Nursing and the Management of Adult Communication Disorders

Contributors

Barbara Aliza, MA, Instructor
Communicative Disorders Department
San Francisco State University
San Francisco, CA
Speech-Language Pathologist
Private Practice
Marin County, CA

Dennis James Arnst, PhD
Audiologist
Veterans Administration Medical Center
San Francisco, CA

Jennifer J. Chiavaras, RN
Head Nurse
Neurobehavior and Aphasia Unit
Boston Veterans Administration
   Medical Center
Boston, MA

Vicky Christianson
Hospital Librarian
Valley Medical Center
Fresno, CA

Chris Hagen, PhD, Director
Speech-Language Pathology
   Department
Speech, Hearing and
   Neurosensory Center
Children's Hospital and Health Center
Sharp Rehabilitation Hospital
San Diego, CA

Nancy Helm-Estabrooks, DSC, Chief
Audiology/Speech Pathology
Boston Veterans Administration
   Medical Center
Assistant Professor of Neurology
   (Speech Pathology)
Boston University School of Medicine
Boston, MA

Karen M. Jensen, MED
Professor of Communicative Disorders
Supervisor, Education of the Deaf
California State University, Fresno
Fresno, CA

Donald L. Mast, MS
Director
Handicapped Students Enabler Program
College of the Sequoias
Visalia, CA

Joyce E. Parker, RN, BSN
Head and Neck Surgery Associates
Suite 780   1633 N. Capitol
Indianapolis, IN 46202

George O. Purvis, PhD
Audiologist
Veterans Administration Medical Center
San Diego, CA
Department of Communicative Disorders
San Diego State University
San Diego, CA

James C. Shanks, PhD
Professor, Speech Pathology
Department of Otolaryngology—Head
   & Neck Surgery
Indiana University School
   of Medicine
Indianapolis, IN

Susan J. Shanks, PhD, Professor
Department of Communicative Disorders
School of Health and Social Work
California State University, Fresno
Fresno, CA

NURSING AND THE MANAGEMENT OF ADULT COMMUNICATION DISORDERS

Editor

Susan J. Shanks, PhD
Professor

California State University, Fresno
Department of Communicative Disorders
School of Health and Social Work

COLLEGE-HILL PRESS, San Diego, California

College-Hill Press, Inc.
4284 41st Street
San Diego, California 92105

Library of Congress Cataloging in Publication Data
Main entry under title:
Nursing and the management of adult communication
   disorders.

   Includes bibliographical references and index.
   1. Communicative disorders—Nursing. I. Shanks,
Susan J., date. [DNLM: 1. Deafness—Nursing texts.
2. Hearing disorders—Nursing texts. 3. Speech disorders—
Nursing texts. 4. Voice disorders—Nursing texts.
5. Language disorders—Nursing texts. WY 158 N9739]
RC423.N87 1983   616.85'5   83–1775
ISBN 0-933014-86-4

Printed in the United States of America

For from him and through him
and to him are all things.
To him be the glory, forever!
Amen.

Romans 11:36
Holy Bible
New International Version

Contents

Preface

The paucity of information for nursing personnel who deal with the communication disorders of adults in acute care and some ambulatory or primary care settings led to the compilation of the chapters for this text. A companion book presents an overview of the management of communication disorders in children.* The contributors to this manuscript, certified communication disorders specialists and their nursing co-authors and consultants, have integrated into eight original chapters those special considerations they feel are necessary in the rehabilitation of adults. The professionals have addressed the needs of patients whose communication disorders are the result of physiological dysfunctioning, the residuals of disease, and progressive conditions; whose functional communication is limited; and or who may never achieve communication proficiency in the oral mode. They have expanded the typical "clinical" plan to the patient's total nursing environment.

Because the book was written for a diverse audience ranging from seasoned professionals to students in training, the contributors have included all essential information to explain the rationale(s) behind the treatment approaches presented and additional references within the text and at the end of each chapter for further study. Appendices with related material also follow several chapters. When possible, illustrations were incorporated to demonstrate how even the smallest gesture and or simplest plan followed by all persons helping the patient may mean the difference between successful communication and confusion.

The audience for this book, in addition to nurses, communication disorders specialists (audiologists, educators of the deaf, and speech-language pathologists), and students in these professions, includes other health personnel who want to help adults who have never had, who are gradually losing, or who have lost the ability to communicate, to maintain their human dignity during and after illness.

Susan J. Shanks

---

*Shanks, S. (Ed.), *Nursing and the Management of Pediatric Communication Disorders*. San Diego: College-Hill Press, 1983.

Foreword

It is better to be sick than to attend the sick. The one is a simple ill; the other combines pain of mind and toil of body.

Euripides: Hippolytus, 428 B.C.[1]

The nurse is no longer delegated to merely carrying out the physician's orders. More than ever it is necessary for the nurse to have a broad general knowledge of all areas of health care and to assume an aggressive, responsible role in initiating health care. This means new skills must be acquired.

This text provides a necessary starting point in the approach to any patient with any communication disorder. Nurses as well as speech-language pathologists, audiologists, educators, and physicians will find this important work extremely helpful in acquiring the background of knowledge to direct the patient with defective communication.

Speech is said to be a picture of the mind. The editor and contributors to this volume focus on a practical clinical approach to speaking problems. The created image forms a solid base for thoughtful panoramic heath care. For the reader the pain of mind in acquiring knowledge is clearly minimized by these authors. Their prior toil and experience imparted herein eases our necessary burden.

Robert L. Calmes, MD

Neurologist
Lecturer, Department of
Communicative Disorders,
California State University,
Fresno
Associate Clinical Professor
of Neurology,
University of California,
Medical Center,
San Francisco

NOTE

[1]Mencken, H.L. *A new dictionary of quotations*. New York: Alfred A. Knopf, 1978, p. 876.

Acknowledgments

This compilation of scholarly chapters is the product of a group of professionals whose cooperation and patience during the editing process were exemplary. My heartfelt thanks are extended to them for making my duties an enriching and pleasurable learning experience.

I am also grateful for the support of each contributor's family and for the stimulation of their colleagues, students, and patients which has led to the formulation of the thoughts found in this book. Deep appreciation is extended to the many readers who have offered suggestions to each of us. To Dennis Arnst, whose initial and continuous enthusiasm prompted many of my efforts during the publishing process, thank you. I am also indebted to Myrthel S. Nelson, RN, MN, CSU Fresno, who encouraged me at critical points, and to Richard D. Ford, Dean, School of Health and Social Work, Sanford M. Brown, Associate Dean, and William M. Coughran, Academic Budget Officer (CSUF) for their support. To Kathy Tanem, who completed many small tasks which cannot be left undone while a book is being edited, thanks. I am also appreciative of the secretarial skills of Bernice Salley and Debi Drew and the continuous assistance, guidance, and encouragement of Kala and S. Singh, our publishers.

Because my initial and subsequent adjustments to quadriplegia (Polio) were positively influenced by my nurse, Grace W. Dawson, at the University of Michigan Hospital who proved to be a vital link in my return to a "normal" life, I dedicate this book to her and to my mother, Martha, who for over 30 years has fulfilled the role of the "ideal, team-oriented" person in my life.

To my many mentors who have provided the examples I needed throughout my professional life, special thanks to you—all.

Susan J. Shanks

1

Communication Disorders Specialists: The Challenge

Susan J. Shanks

During the past decade training programs in the allied health professions have developed a closer relationship between nurses, communication disorders (CD) specialists, and other health professionals involved in management of adults with health problems. However, training focus has not provided wide exposure to or experience with the communication disorders of adults. Nursing professionals may enter the work setting eager to cooperate during the treatment process but ill-prepared for the collaboration desired by the communication disorders specialist. Therefore, in most health settings, on-the-job continuing education has been necessary before nurses could become maximally involved in treatment programs for the adult with a communication disorder. To be adequately prepared for collaboration, nurses should have a core of knowledge about communication disorders, and about the rehabilitation of patients with these disorders and associated complications. In this book rehabilitation will refer to the process of developing a person's communication to the best possible functioning level.

This book will introduce the reader to the communication disorders most commonly found in the adult population and will provide programming suggestions for nurses and others who care for these patients. The goals of certain patients with communication disorders cannot be achieved without the cooperation of all CD specialists. This chapter will describe the CD professionals and delineate the special qualifications of these persons who play such an important role in the rehabilitation of our target population.

The various titles utilized by CD specialists may be confusing to other health professionals. The specialist who diagnoses and carries out a treatment program for the patient who has a speech, voice, and or language disorder is a *speech-language pathologist* (SLP), but may also be called a speech clinician; a speech correctionist; or a speech therapist (Bloodstein, 1979; Perkins, 1971). Because the term "therapist" is not considered to be reflective of the ability to work independently of medical supervision or referral, the title speech therapist has been avoided by members of the American Speech-Language-Hearing Association (ASHA). SLPs who provide clinical services in any setting can be recognized professionally by obtaining the Certificate of Clinical Competence (CCC–Speech-Language pathology) from ASHA. Thirty-two states require a state license for SLPs to practice in non-public agencies.

The CD specialist who diagnoses hearing losses, makes medical referrals, cooperates with physicians in differential diagnosis of health problems and or recommends hearing aids is called an *audiologist.* In most health settings audiologists must have national certification from ASHA (CCC–Audiology) or a state license to practice. When warranted audiologists also plan and implement aural rehabilitation programs which include care and use of a hearing aid and lipreading skills.

Audiologists work closely with *educators of the deaf* who have the primary responsibility for the education of deaf students. The counseling and interpreting roles of these educators continue to be important to the deaf adult. Educators of the deaf often assume teaching roles in high schools and community college programs for the handicapped, and are responsible for most sign language courses being offered through various community agencies. Rehabilitation programs and recreation agencies also rely on the educator of the deaf to provide services to deaf adults. More lengthy discussions of the specific contributions of these CD specialists as they work with the nurse and the adult with communication disorders and associated problems are found in the chapters which follow.

Nurses can be significant liaisons for deaf patients seeking health care. Anyone who has heard a deaf adult relate the numerous communication breakdowns and successes which take place throughout his or her life knows that this communication disordered population offers a special challenge and requires much skill of the health professional. Working with the adult who has acquired a communication disorder also presents a stimulating challenge to all involved. These patients have a different perspective of the communicative process and often have less patience with their inability to communicate partially or totally than the person who has suffered from a problem since childhood. The chapters which follow describe how we, the helping professionals, can meet this challenge as we cooperate to understand this perspective and plan together to incorporate the unique needs of each adult into our assessment and treatment programs.

REFERENCES

Bloodstein, O. *Speech pathology: An introduction.* Boston: Houghton Mifflin Co., 1979.

Perkins, W.H. *Speech pathology: An applied behavioral science.* St. Louis: C.V. Mosby Co., 1971.

2

The Nurse and Voice Disorders

Joyce E. Parker
James C. Shanks

INTRODUCTION

Verbalizing one's thoughts is a major expression of self and personality. A voice disorder which impairs the exchange of conversation and ideas can create a sense of isolation. Whether a person has been reserved or outspoken, loss of natural voice is a threat to self-esteem and image. The nurse who is alert to this psychological difficulty can assist the patient with a voice disorder in dealing with the problem.

Nurses may encounter patients with voice disorders in almost any aspect of practice. Voice disorders can affect the healthy male and female of any age, race, geographic location, or socioeconomic level and can compound problems for the ill person. This chapter will explain how the nurse can play an important role in the rehabilitation of adults with voice disorders.

Special Nursing Skills/Knowledge

Acute care nurses who meet patients with voice disorders for the first time will find some special skills are required to work with this population. The nurse can cushion the impact of the loss of voice by creating an atmosphere of trust when the patient and family members are initially seen. After taking a thorough case history, the nurse can explain ordered tests and forthcoming treatments, if needed, in understandable terms to relieve anxiety about the condition, and to prepare the patient for future referrals.

Educating the patient and family members about the importance of correct vocal habits is often the task of the nurse. Many vocal disorders may be prevented and or improved by a change in vocal habits. The nurse can monitor and reinforce the prescribed hygiene regime.

Vocal Hygiene

Nurses can structure the vocal hygiene program by first managing the environment of the patient for maximum vocal mechanism health. In the hospital a bedside humidifier can be useful in delivering moisture to irritated mucous membranes of the respiratory tract and in liquefying thick secretions. Beyond such action by the nurse in the hospital, vocal hygiene can take many directions. From a variety of sources, Wilson (1979) culled many suggestions for patients. The following are representative:

1. Avoid loud talking, shouting, laughing, cheering, or singing. These activities should be shunned, whether undertaken in jest, anger, demonstration, in noise, or to accommodate hearing impaired people.
2. Seek easier closure of the vocal folds in coughing, throat clearing, lifting, grunting, and sneezing.
3. Try to begin voice more softly, more gently, and more easily, without undue strain, glottal attack, or abruptness.
4. Breathe air which is humidified, filtered, and of moderate temperature, if possible.

Voice rest is often prescribed for some vocal fold problems and after diagnostic procedures such as direct or fiberoptic laryngoscopy. Prolonged voice rest may be a source of anxiety for the patient and family. Voice rest may vary from complete silence for a specified time to the limited use of the voice for a period of several weeks. The nurse can introduce alternative means of nonoral communication, described in Chapter 8 of this book, to help the patient through this time of stress. Compliance may increase if the nurse explains the consequences of speaking, further injury to the larynx or prolongation of the problem. The call light in the nursing unit or a small bell placed within the patient's reach in the home may help allay fears of being unable to call vocally for help. Patients who have a normal laryngeal structure might use an electrolarynx to offset vocalization attempts.

For further discussion of vocal hygiene procedures see Brodnitz (1967), Cooper (1973), and Wilson (1979).

Overview of Nursing Responsibilities

The nurse's role is most important in the pre- and post-operative care of the patient with voice problems. Preoperative nursing responsibilities include teaching the patient the steps followed in diagnosis, nutritional assessment, and the maintenance of good oral hygiene. Psychological preparation of the patient and or family unit regarding the anticipated surgery should include discussion of the procedure and post-op equipment, such as drains, nasogastric tubes, and so on. Questions regarding post-op appearance and the individual's ability to speak and swallow should be dealt with as extensively as the patient desires. When appropriate, multidisciplinary team referrals may be made to social workers, occupational therapists, physical therapists, speech-language pathologists, and chaplainsy.

Postoperatively, the maintenance of a patent airway is of highest priority and often the most demanding of nursing responsibilities. The patient should be encouraged to cough effectively to clear the airway and help prevent atelectasis and or pneumonia. When a tracheostomy is present and coughing is ineffective, suctioning of the secretions must be done as often as necessary. Other immediate post-op care is focused on wound care, mouth care, balance of fluid and electrolytes, plus general patient comfort. Nursing goals include keeping the patient free from preventable complications, minimizing pain and discomfort, and providing emotional support.

Discharge planning is a multidisciplinary effort, utilizing all team members to attain an adequate level of patient self-care. Family involvement also can smooth the transition from the hospital to the home setting. Follow-up treatment and therapy as well as referrals to community services that provide home health care also may be arranged through the team.

Before considering specific vocal disorders, it is appropriate to review the nature of the structure and function of the laryngeal mechanism in voice production. To better participate in treatment protocol, the nurse needs to be knowledgeable of the structure and function of the upper airway and food passages in relation to normal and problem voice production. Consideration of the normal highlights discussion of the abnormal.

See Moore (1971) for the nature of, and Weinberg (1971) for the sound of, voice disorders.

The Normal Larynx

The larynx, or "voice-box," is composed of three paired and three unpaired cartilages, held together by muscles and ligaments. Connecting the

pharynx with the trachea, the stiff cartilaginous, laryngeal framework pro-
tects the vocal folds and permits an airway. The true vocal folds, which are
folds of mucous membrane, work systematically with other laryngeal structures to open and close the airway during inspiration and expiration. Closure
of the glottis, or space between the vocal folds, permits voluntary increase of
intrathoracic pressure. Without closure of the glottis, cough would be weak
and inefficient. Opening the glottis is essential to permit respiration and
adequate exchange of gases necessary to life.

The larynx is innervated by the Xth cranial or vagus nerve. The recurrent
laryngeal nerve, a branch of the vagus, is responsible for most of the motor
nerve supply of the larynx. The superior laryngeal nerve affords the sensory
nerve supply of the larynx and the motor nerve supply for the tensor of the
vocal folds, the cricothyroid muscle.

The lymphatic system of the larynx drains to lymph nodes in the middle
and upper cervical chain along the internal jugular vein of the neck. This is an
important consideration when dealing with laryngeal malignancies because
metastatic cells spread along lymphatic channels.

Another major laryngeal function is to allow for phonation, defined as
voice, a physiologic process in which moving air is converted into acoustic
energy (Zemlin, 1968). A delicate coordination between the muscles of the
larynx, expired air flow, musculature of the pharynx, soft palate, tongue,
and lips is necessary to achieve normal voice. Any upset in the balanced
coordination of muscles, nerves, and psychological perception of voice can
affect the desired output of the system—voice/speech production. The result
can be a voice disorder.

VOICE DISORDERS

Age-Related Voice Disorders

Disordered phonation may be present as early as the birth cry. Congenital
or neonatal conditions have been reported as providing distinctive sounds
which may provide clues to diagnosis of a threat to health.

A premature infant may present a weak cry. The weakness may stem from
hypotonia or lack of muscle tone associated with Down's syndrome or tri-
somy 21 syndrome. An infant with a vascular ring, a cardiovascular anomaly,
may have a very soft cry due to expiratory obstruction from the compressed
trachea and esophagus. Disordered voice may be overshadowed by respiration in disorders such as croup, cystic fibrosis, hyaline membrane disease,
asthma, whooping cough, or pneumonia. An unusually low-pitched voice
may be associated with hypothyroidism, precocious puberty, or virilization

of the female voice. A hoarse voice may result from lipoid proteinosis as well as the more common finding of laryngitis, regardless of age.

For a review of the aging process and voice disorders see Meyerson and Shanks (1981).

Laryngitis

Laryngitis may exist in both chronic and acute phases. Causes range from bacterial and viral infectious agents to trauma from irritants such as smoking, alcohol ingestion, and voice abuse. Common symptoms include hoarseness, pain, and cough. Treatment is directed by the cause: Appropriate medication for infectious agents and removal of the irritant in traumatic cases. Generalized upper respiratory infections with laryngitis are treated systemically.

Localized acute infections of the larynx may occur at any age. In the adult (and even more often in the infant) acute epiglotitis can cause rapid and extreme dyspnea. Establishment of an adequate airway by endotracheal entubation or tracheostomy may be necessary while the antibiotic regime is initiated and followed.

The treatment regime is enhanced by environmental supports such as high humidity. Suggestions of nonverbal communication patterns rather than verbal communication may be given to allow for voice rest, a common treatment for laryngitis.

Laryngeal Trauma

A patent airway is also of primary importance in patients experiencing trauma. The most frequent cause of injury to the larynx is the blunt-trauma blow sustained to the neck, such as that associated with auto accidents. Subcutaneous emphysema is a symptom indicative of a possible laryngeal fracture. Tears in the mucous membrane lining of the larynx may induce rapid accumulation of fluid or blood that can also produce an acute laryngeal obstruction. Fractures and dislocations of the laryngeal cartilages compound the airway obstruction.

Continued assessment of the airway is critical to monitor patency and adequate air exchange. Symptoms of increased respiration and pulse rates, cyanosis, increasing dyspnea and or stridor, deformities in neck contour, and restlessness are indications that the natural airway is in jeopardy and that a tracheostomy may be necessary. Endoscopy equipment as well as instruments to do a tracheostomy should be available for use.

Vocal Nodules

Sometimes called "singer's nodes," vocal nodules are benign growths that result from voice misuse or abuse. They appear as reddened, raised lesions to the examiner, and usually are noted at the juncture of the anterior one-third and posterior two-thirds of the true vocal folds. Due to the inability of the folds to achieve good approximation, the voice sounds hoarse to the listener. Conservative treatment includes voice therapy to improve voice use and habits. If surgical removal is necessary, care should be taken to remove only the nodule and not part of the vocal fold, which could produce a more permanent change in voice quality. Because voice rest should be observed following surgery for removal of a vocal nodule, the nurse should encourage the patient to use the nonverbal means of communication mentioned above.

See K. Wilson (1979) for discussion of treatment of vocal nodules.

Laryngeal Polyps

Laryngeal polyps may be attached to the vocal fold by a narrow or broad base, or may hang on a pedicle of mucous membrane near the vocal fold. The polyp, an edematous mass of mucous membrane, may move with respiration. Symptoms of hoarseness or other voice change may warrant surgical removal.

Papillomatosis

Papilloma may present to both juvenile and adult patients. Believed to be viral in nature, the florid growth of the grayish white, cluster-like papilloma may severely compromise the airway and necessitate a tracheostomy for adequate air exchange. Symptoms range from mild hoarseness to total loss of voice, e.g. aphonia. Papilloma may occur throughout the larynx, including the trachea and epiglottis, but are more commonly noted on the true vocal fold. Juvenile papilloma tend to subside at puberty.

Treatment is necessary to maintain a patent airway. Due to their recurrent tendencies, repeated removals are not uncommon. Surgical removal, via direct laryngoscopy utilizing cup forceps to manually excise the papilloma, is a well-known treatment, although other treatment modalities utilize the carbon dioxide laser, cryotherapy, ultrasonic techniques, and topical chemotherapy.

Laryngeal Paralysis

Disease or injury of either the superior or recurrent laryngeal nerves may result in paralysis as diagnosed by observation of vocal fold movement upon direct or indirect examination. This may be a sequela of thyroid surgery. Injury or disease of the vagus nerve may affect motor and or sensory branch functions. Examination using a laryngeal mirror or direct observation may show a paralyzed vocal fold unable to properly abduct from the median or paramedian position. Symptoms of hoarseness or breathiness depend, in part, on compensation by the opposite fold. If the nonparalyzed fold moves to the midline and beyond to approximate the paralyzed fold, there may be little breathiness. Hoarseness, a combination of breathiness and tension of the larynx, is perceived when the folds are unable to close the glottis. The resulting air escape contributes to turbulence and asymmetric fold vibration.

Unilateral fold paralysis may be left untreated if compensatory action of the nonparalyzed fold is adequate. Surgical-grade Teflon paste is sometimes injected into the flaccid paralyzed fold to augment the fold and push it toward the midline. This allows for better fold approximation and better voice, sometimes at the expense of pulmonary ventilation with a reduced airway.

Bilateral fold paralysis is rare. If both folds are in the median position, the airway may be significantly compromised, even to the point of necessitating a tracheostomy. Treatment is first aimed at restoration of the airway, rather than voice improvement.

Elective Mutism

There are some conditions in which voluntary function of vocal fold adduction/abduction is missing due to paralysis. In others, the voluntary function appears to be missing despite absence of paralysis. In the latter condition, the patient has voice in one environment or set of circumstances (such as home), yet has no voice at another time or place. It is as though the person elects times in which to be mute because of some psychosocial problem. This elective mutism may be seen as a defense against an environment perceived to be hostile or threatening. In this condition, the person still retains the abililty to control the laryngeal mechanism for nonphonatory functions, such as coughing, even when voiceless. These functions hold the clue to another condition in which the speaker seems to completely lose the function of voicing.

Hysterical Aphonia

A related psychosocial condition in which the speaker seems to totally lose the ability to voice is called hysterical aphonia. Communication may be whispered, yet the patient is aphonic. However, the nonorganic nature of "hysterical aphonia" is discerned when the patient unwittingly approximates and controls the vocal folds in throat clearing and coughing.

Management of elective mutism and hysterical aphonia may include emotional support of the person and, without confrontation or challenge which might imply criticism, clinical treatment suggesting that voice which is present during coughing can return. The nurse can reinforce the person's efforts to regain voice at a symptom level while not engendering guilt at a deeper level.

For a description of these disorders read Aronson (1980).

Registers

At times the nurse may hear a voice which sounds like bacon frying in a skillet. This distinctive quality usually occurs at the end of a word or at the end of a sentence. If used extensively, it conveys the impression of an older, perhaps infirm, person. Although the condition does not imply laryngeal pathology, its user may benefit from referral for voice therapy designed to raise the flow of air and or the pitch.

A voice which is pitched inappropriately high may result from a smaller than average larynx. If the vocal folds are of average size for the speaker's age and sex, the high-pitched voice may be identified as a falsetto voice. A person may use the falsetto mechanism intentionally, as in singing popular music. However, its use on an involuntary basis may signal faulty learning. At puberty, the growth of vocal folds and the resulting lowering of fundamental frequency or pitch may be masked as the person habitually shifts into the falsetto posture. Generally, this voice is a bit softer and does not project or carry well.

Correction of involuntary falsetto involves three steps: (1) identification of the normal (modal) voice, (2) habituation, and (3) acceptance of the normal voice. Finding the lower voice may spring from coughing, throat clearing, holding the larynx down digitally, pulling the larynx down by hyperextending the head back, or forcing a loud voice to jar more vocal fold mass into vibration.

Managing persons with voice disorders can involve more than voice therapy techniques alone. Nursing cooperation in humidification of vocal folds, either by altering environmental air or by stimulating ventricular secretions, may be beneficial. As noted above, vocal abuses or misuses need to be identified and reduced in an effort to provide healthy vocal fold tissue. Indeed, some programs of voice therapy are built around the reduction of faulty vocal habits. Other programs stress positive action— what to do—as opposed to negative steps of what not to do.

Boone (1977) has outlined 24 specific voice therapy techniques speech-language pathologists use to facilitate voice or vocal fold function.

Many of these specific disorders discussed above affect the vibrating source of the voice, the vocal folds, that in turn, change the features (parameters) of voice identified as pitch, loudness, and quality (with time as a related factor). In addition to voice disorders associated with psycho-social problems and benign laryngeal pathology, laryngeal malignancies may cause dysphonia, voice disorders, or aphonia, complete and permanent loss of voice.

LARYNGEAL MALIGNANCIES

While squamous cell carcinoma is the principal laryngeal malignancy, other epithelial and nonepithelial tumors also occur in the larynx. Laryngeal carcinoma represents less than 1% of malignant lesions. It has been estimated that the incidence of laryngeal carcinoma is one new case per 100,000 population (Batsakis, 1974). According to statistics it is more common in men. The male-to-female ratio generally cited is 10:1, although the incidence of laryngeal cancer in females is increasing. As observed by Wynder (1975), the sex ratio of occurrence of laryngeal cancer was 14.9:1 in 1956, increasing to 4.6:1 in 1973. The peak ages for occurrence are the 6th and 7th decades, with the majority of cases occurring between the ages of 40 and 69.

In some studies investigating occupations and the occurrence of laryngeal cancer, no correlation was found. However, other investigators reported an increased incidence in persons who had been exposed to asbestos. Prior exposure to radiation and certain dietary factors in various cultures also have been cited as factors increasing susceptibility to laryngeal cancer. Epidemiologic studies have implicated cigarette smoking more than alcohol use as a causal factor in the development of this disease. Lowry (1975) noted a strong association between heavy alcoholic intake and development of cancer of the supraglottic larynx, though not of the vocal folds.

Symptoms of a laryngeal malignancy vary, depending on the exact structures involved with the tumor and the size of the tumor. If the true vocal fold is the primary site, the initial symptom of hoarseness can lead to an early diagnosis. Any patient whose hoarseness persists longer than 2 weeks should have a laryngeal examination.

Subjective symptoms develop more slowly with tumors involving parts of the larynx other than the true vocal folds. Complaints of dysphagia, problems with swallowing, voice changes, a burning pain when swallowing, painless neck nodes, and dyspnea should be investigated. Besides documentation of subjective symptoms, smoking and alcohol consumption habits should be included when taking the patient's history.

Diagnosis of laryngeal cancer is made from evaluations of subjective and objective symptoms and from a biopsy of the involved area. Direct laryngoscopy is performed not only to obtain a small biopsy for the pathology lab to analyze, but also to determine the extent of the lesion for proper staging and selection of a treatment modality.

The type of treatment recommended is determined by the exact tumor location, its stage of development, the presence or absence of neck node metastases, or other distant metastases (such as bone, liver, spleen, or lungs). The patient's general condition, including age, nutritional status, and personal desires are also taken into consideration.

In general, an early laryngeal lesion of the true folds responds successfully to radiation therapy or a limited surgical procedure. More extensive tumors require surgery and radiation therapy, singly, or in combination. Chemotherapy and immunotherapy hold promise for being important adjuncts to the treatment course. The nurse can help the patient accept the protocol by answering questions about the treatment itself and by explaining anticipated changes, thus, better preparing the patient for surgery or radiation therapy. An attitude of compassion without pity and optimism without false hope can help the nurse support and care for the patient and family unit throughout stressful periods or crises.

Along with the goal of complete tumor removal, optimal treatment includes better patient rehabilitation following surgery. Recent advances in head and neck oncology are significantly improving the outlook on rehabilitation.

Partial Laryngectomy

Hemilaryngectomy. In patients with limited tumor involvement affecting only one vocal fold, a hemilaryngectomy may be the treatment of choice. Also termed a *vertical laryngectomy* due to the vertical incision in the middle of the neck, approximately one half of the larynx is resected including the diseased true fold, ventricle, and false vocal fold. Conservation laryngeal surgery represents an important advance in head and neck oncology, allowing for preservation of the laryngeal functions of swallowing and phonation without compromising the curability of the disease.

Preoperatively, the patient is assessed and prepared for surgery in ways which have been discussed previously. The patient should understand that a temporary tracheostomy will be present postoperatively. The tracheostomy bypasses the edematous surgical site and allows for proper tissue healing in the remaining larynx. Secretions must be suctioned from the tracheostomy as needed to assure a patent airway. Phonation is difficult without occlusion of the tracheostomy tube; therefore, an alternative means of communication should be provided.

Postoperatively, patients are fed through nasogastric tubes for about 1 week to facilitate healing of the remaining larynx. Swallowing may be difficult at first, due to glottic edema. Initial oral feedings following surgery should be closely monitored for aspiration. When adequate swallowing function has been reestablished, gradual decannulation (removal of the trach tube) is achieved over a period of 3 to 5 days.

Supraglottic Laryngectomy. For carcinoma of the epiglottis and adjacent structures above the level of the true fold, a supraglottic or *horizontal laryngectomy* represents another conservation procedure aimed at preservation of normal laryngeal function. The upper portion of the larynx is removed via a horizontal incision just above the true vocal folds which leaves the folds, themselves, intact. If metastases to the lymph nodes in the neck are noted, a radical neck dissection also is performed.

For a patient having a supraglottic laryngectomy, the road to rehabilitation requires patience to preserve normal laryngeal functions of swallowing and phonation. Full support of the multidisciplinary team will enhance rehabilitation. Because of the surgical removal of the epiglottis and false folds, foods and liquids taken orally tend to spill directly into the trachea. Aspiration may pose a problem which can delay patient rehabilitation and tracheal decannulation.

Preoperative considerations emphasize the need for patient and family awareness of expected postoperative equipment, including tracheostomy, nasogastric tube, drainage tubes, dressings, and so on. The need to spend the first postoperative night in an intensive care setting should be anticipated and explained. Nonverbal communication patterns for use after surgery should be agreed on preoperatively. Patient questions regarding appearance and abilities should be answered honestly and tactfully.

For the patient undergoing a supraglottic laryngectomy, a tracheostomy is mandatory inasmuch as surgical changes and edema do not permit an adequate airway. The use of a cuffed trach tube that can be alternately inflated and deflated is important in diminishing aspiration. Special attention is given to deflating the cuff at scheduled intervals. This allows for suctioning of secretions which have spilled from the pharynx into the trachea and prevents tracheal erosion. As healing occurs, the cuff is deflated for longer periods of time. The ultimate goal of decannulation is dependent on the patient relearning to swallow.

Postoperatively, the patient is fed for a minimum of 10 to 14 days with a nasogastric tube. Cautious oral feedings of semisolid foods are initiated with close monitoring for symptoms of aspiration, which include coughing of "swallowed" food, evidence of food at the trach site, cyanosis, or unexplained tachycardia. Relearning how to swallow includes directing the patient to maintain an upright, sitting position. To facilitate closure of the glottis during swallowing, the patient should be instructed to hold his or her breath. After swallowing several times, the patient is instructed to cough. Any aspirated feeding will be coughed up through the tracheostomy tube or into the oral cavity. Relearning the swallowing process can be a frustrating task for both the patient and the nurse. Frequent repetition of instructions combined with an unhurried, encouraging attitude by the nurse can do much to enhance the rehabilitation of the patient. For further information on dealing with swallowing problems, see Chapter 7 of this book.

If the relearning of swallowing has not been achieved prior to discharge, the patient may be maintained on enteral therapy at home. Patients and families need information and practice to learn the use, care, and maintenance of the nasogastric tube. A dietician may be helpful in counseling the family on diet and food selection.

Following decannulation, the voice is usually of normal tone and quality. Complications or difficulties with swallowing with tracheal decannulation tend to occur in proportion to the extent of the supraglottic resection, as well as the age and general medical condition of the patient (Lawson & Biller, 1981).

Total Laryngectomy

Total laryngectomy is the treatment reserved for patients with advanced carcinoma of the true folds, i.e., tumors which have shown invasion of cartilages of the larynx, fixation of cord mobility, or tumors which have spread beyond the larynx into the hypopharynx, or base of the tongue. Patients with conditions such as advanced age, debility, and chronic pulmonary disease, factors that would jeopardize patient relearning of the swallowing process, are also considered for total laryngectomy. This procedure eliminates problems of postoperative aspiration.

Total laryngectomy includes removal of the thyroid cartilage, hyoid bone, cricoid cartilage, and part of the trachea. If the disease has extended into the neck or lymph system, a radical neck dissection also may be necessary. The

FIGURE 2–1
Before total laryngectomy

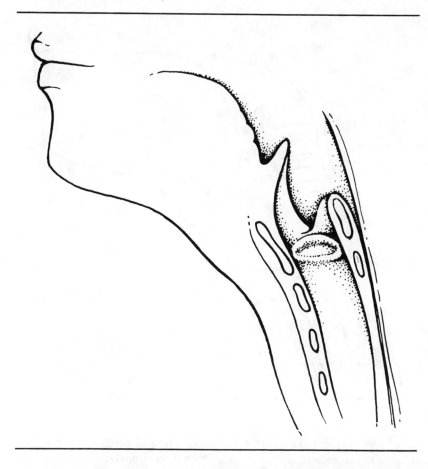

complete removal of the larynx mandates creation of a permanent tracheostomy to provide for an airway. This is done by suturing the remaining trachea to the skin of the lower neck. The mouth and nose no longer are part of the pulmonary airway. Still connected to the esophagus, the mouth and nose maintain their functions as part of the alimentary tract and allow the patient to eat by mouth. However, all air exchange is through the neck stoma. Patients are now neck breathers. Smell and taste after surgery are diminished due to the change in the breathing pathway. (See Figures 2–1, 2–2.) Although removing the larynx eliminates laryngeal phonation, substitute voice can be acquired.

Nursing responsibilities for the patient undergoing total laryngectomy present multiple challenges, and require the nurse to draw on a broad base of

FIGURE 2–2

After total laryngectomy

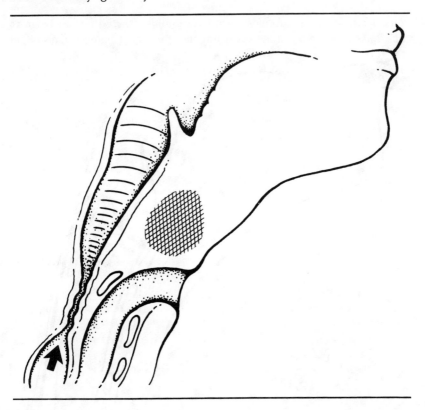

knowledge. Besides caring for the obvious physical needs, the nurse also must be cognizant and alert to the less obvious emotional needs and psychosocial changes being faced by the patient/family unit.

On admission to the hospital, the nurse should begin to assess the patient's symptoms, health habits, occupation, living conditions, and support systems. As insight is gained, the nurse is better able to understand the patient's ability to accept his or her disease, the planned therapeutic intervention, and expected postoperative changes such as loss of voice. Asking the patient what the doctor has said and about surgery will help in evaluating his or her mental and emotional state. A trusting relationship established preoperatively between the nurse and patient/family unit can greatly enhance the postoperative course and rehabilitation period.

Studies have shown that, preoperatively, patients and families have felt inadequately informed (Gonnella, Parker, Hollender, Lowell, Petterson, &

Miller, 1978). Many times the role of informant falls on the nurse. By interpreting information given by the physician to the patient, the nurse may help the patient understand the treatment course and correct any misconceptions. Understanding complex information allows the patient to begin to cope and to ventilate feelings regarding the anticipated changes in his or her life.

Each patient is an individual with unique coping skills and support systems. By interacting with the patient, the nurse can reinforce positive coping skills and help the patient identify nonproductive coping techniques. The patient may display emotions of anger, denial, and depression as mechanisms of coping. Each rehabilitation program should be individually tailored to meet the patient/family unit's needs. Multidisciplinary referrals by the nurse can provide the necessary information and support. Preparing the patient and family psychologically for surgery and its expected outcomes should not be underestimated or overlooked.

Other possible sources of anxiety to both the patient and family include dealing with the results of anatomic changes after laryngectomy. Changes include loss of normal laryngeal voice, breathing through a neck stoma, alterations in taste and in smell, and changes in normal breathing and coughing patterns. Such changes have an impact in both physiological function and body image as noted by Fisher (1970).

Consequences of a total laryngectomy, including altered communication skills and activities of daily living, may jeopardize the patient's job, career goals, family structure, and role in society. Threatened changes in self-esteem and self-worth may be even more devastating than the disease process.

"Cancer" continues to be a word associated with pain, mutilation, and death. By offering acceptance without fostering unrealistic expectations of postoperative abilities, the rehabilitation team can guide the patient towards hope and optimal independence.

Equally important, patient education regarding postoperative physical needs should be initiated by the rehabilitation team prior to surgery. As discussed in earlier sections, postoperative equipment, including drains, dressings, tracheostomy tube, and nasogastric tube should be explained. A means of nonverbal communication ought to be selected. The nurse must reassure the patient that he or she will be checked frequently following surgery, that measures to control pain will be instituted, and that assistance with every aspect of care will be provided.

A preoperative visit by a speech-language pathologist is often helpful to introduce the patient to alternatives to laryngeal speech. Discussion of these alternatives is presented in the following section. This interview allows the clinician to assess the patient's speaking and hearing status before surgery.

Preoperatively, a patient may benefit from meeting a person who has already been laryngectomized. Local chapters of the American Cancer

Society or International Association of Laryngectomees (IAL), often known as Lost Chord or New Voice Clubs, can provide volunteers to visit the patient and family. However, each patient presents an individual attitude. What may be a satisfying and encouraging preop visit for one patient may only reinforce disaster to another. Each situation requires thoughtful evaluation and leadership from the primary physician. In most cases, the patient should share in making the final decision regarding meeting with a person who has had a laryngectomy.

The postoperative nursing care of a patient having a total laryngectomy is a challenge requiring specialized training and astute observation. An intensive care setting frequently is utilized to facilitate airway maintenance, wound management, and fluid balance, as well as to minimize complications following surgery and general anesthesia.

Initially, airway maintenance requires the most demanding care, as each patient has a newly created tracheostoma. Keeping the airway free of secretions requires frequent suctioning of the trachea and stoma if the patient is unable to effectively cough and expel the secretions by him or herself. A metal or plastic laryngectomy tube may be used to maintain stoma size and enhance pulmonary toilet. The initial tube change is the physician's responsibility. To keep the airway patent, the inner cannula of the tube should be removed, cleaned, and replaced as frequently as necessary. Responsibility for such care can be transferred gradually from the nurse to the patient.

As the normal airway has been surgically altered, the sinuses, which usually warm, filter, and humidify inspired air, have been bypassed. Humidity must be added to the patient's environment to reduce irritation of tracheal mucous membranes and to liquefy thick secretions. Frequently, humidity is delivered by a trach collar immediately postop and by a bedside humidifier during convalescence. Installing a few drops of sterile normal saline directly into the stoma helps loosen crusts and moistens irritated tracheal membranes. If humidity is not added, crusts harden and adhere to the tracheal wall, causing further tracheal irritation and bleeding. Mucous plugs, collections of hardened mucous and secretions, must be removed from the stoma area and upper trachea using blunt forceps or a hemostat. A plug, once allowed to form, can increase rapidly in size by the adherence of more mucous and can shift in position within the trachea when the patient coughs. A mucous plug can completely occlude the patient's airway, requiring urgent action to reestablish airway patency. Aggressive suctioning, changing of the entire laryngectomy tube, instillation of 3 to 5 mls of normal saline, and patient coughing are helpful in coping with mucous plugs. The best defense against mucous plugs is prevention, utilizing scrupulous routine observation, plus care of the stoma and trachea.

Wound observation and care following total laryngectomy is also of critical importance. Some physicians choose to apply large pressure dressings following surgery which must be observed for excessive drainage. Other physicians elect not to dress the wound, which allows for easier observation of the skin flaps and incision lines. Drains placed during surgery require sufficient suctioning pressure to keep the wound skin flaps flattened, to show drainage movement in the tubing toward the drain reservoir, and to keep the reservoir itself compressed. If no dressings are present, observation for swelling under the skin flaps must be made. Signs of swelling include an increase in flap edema, change in skin coloration or blanching, change in the type or rate of drainage, or airway compression. In addition, changes in hemoglobin and hematocrit levels consistent with blood loss may indicate a hematoma is forming within the wound. The surgeon should be notified at once if this is suspected. Further surgery may be required to stop the bleeding.

Other wound complications include excessive tissue edema, which may be decreased with proper positioning. The head of the bed should be elevated approximately 45 degrees and the patient should avoid sleeping on the operated side to prevent accumulation of fluid.

Development of an unplanned fistula is another complication prolonging hospitalization and slowing recovery. A chyle fistula is the result of lymphatic system leak, and is often noted due to the amount and consistency of drainage in the drain system. Chyle may be clear or milky white, unlike the expected serosanguinous wound drainage. Development of a fistula which leaks saliva indicates a breakdown in the closure of the pharynx. Saliva swallowed by the patient leaks through the defect and eventually through the overlying neck skin, creating a pharyngocutaneous fistula. Fistulae formation predisposes the patient to infection, skin maceration, and tracheal soiling. Treatment includes feeding the patient by a nasogastric tube to avoid further stress on the pharyngeal defect. Medicated packing may be used to facilitate closure of the fistula from within the wound. Small, pinpoint fistulae may close spontaneously in a few days or weeks, while larger ones may require months or even further surgery to close.

Rupture of the carotid artery, sometimes termed a carotid blow-out, is a potentially grave complication noted more frequently in patients having undergone a radical neck dissection. Carotid ruptures occur more frequently in the presence of: wound breakdown, fistula, necrosis, tissues treated with radiation therapy, and loss of a flap or vessel exposure. A slight trickle of blood may herald an imminent rupture, which may occur from days to weeks postoperatively. If bleeding does occur, immediate, firm, and constant pressure should be applied while additional help is summoned. Supplies (a cuffed tracheotomy tube, hemostats, adequate suction equipment, a cut-down tray to start an intravenous, IV administration sets and solutions, and packing) kept at the patient's bedside may save precious seconds in time of a true vascular emergency.

Other postoperative nursing intervention includes maintenance of good nutrition, vital to tissue healing. The total laryngectomy patient will receive feedings via a nasogastric tube for 7 to 10 days postoperatively to prevent breakdown of the pharyngeal suture line which reduces subsequent fistula formation. Soft foods will be introduced gradually at first, shifting toward solid foods and regular diet as progress is made.

When strength and confidence are gained, the patient should be encouraged to partake in self care, including tube feedings, stoma care and suctioning, oral hygiene, and recording of intake and output of fluids. Demonstration by the nurse to the patient, written instructions, and a return demonstration by the patient back to the nurse will help the patient/family unit learn new methods of care. Hannahs, Hooper, and Sigler (1981) provide detailed information on nursing care of patients with surgery of the head and neck area. Baker and Cunningham (1980) give a helpful overview of vocal rehabilitation for laryngectomees. Added details follow.

POST-LARYNGECTOMY COMMUNICATION

Postoperative communication centers on the patient's loss of laryngeal phonation. Immediately after surgery, language to convey needs may be expressed best by writing, gesturing, or by pointing to printed words or pictures. Gradually this mode of language expression is replaced by an artificial larynx, by esophageal voice, or by a surgically facilitated voice.

Artificial Larynx

The manufactured larynx requires a power source to create sound. There are two primary sources of power: air and electricity.

Pneumatic devices use air to activate or vibrate substances as varied as a rubber band, a metal reed, or a pitch pipe. Electrical devices use batteries to activate materials such as pistons or solid discs (see Figure 2–3, 2–4).

Sound so generated must be conducted into the vocal tract, more commonly known as the throat and or mouth. Sound introduced into the vocal tract can be resonated and articulated, e.g., formed into vowels and consonants for words of connected speech. An artificial larynx which utilizes pulmonary air power serves to connect the stoma, through which air is expelled, to the mouth, the entrance to the vocal tract. A battery-powered electrolarynx can deliver sound through the wall of the neck, through the cheek, or directly into the mouth via a tube.

FIGURE 2-3
Electrolarynx

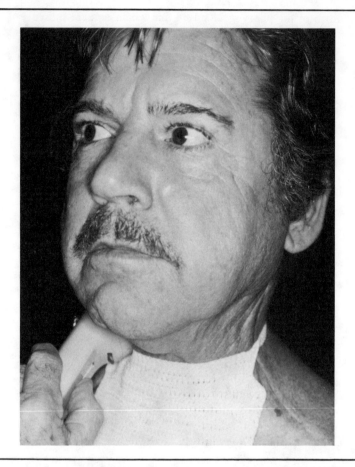

See Diedrich and Youngstrom (1966) for descriptions of artificial larynxes.

The following suggestions may be helpful to the nurse assisting the patient to communicate more effectively with the artificial larynx. The nurse can make sure that sound is channeled effectively from the instrument head into the neck wall, that tone is sustained throughout each natural phrase, and that the articulators (lips, tongue, jaw) are moved enough to produce distinctive speech sounds.

FIGURE 2–4
Mechanical larynx

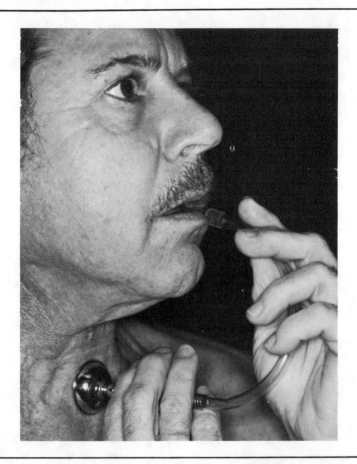

More important than technique is the attitude concerning use of the artificial larynx. In recent years there has been a considerable shift toward the early and enthusiastic use of the artificial larynx. Using an artificial larynx enables the patient to resume speaking soon after surgery. Articulation skills used with an instrument to maintain preop skills are transferred to esophageal speech. Even when esophageal speech is developed, the artificial larynx is helpful under various conditions: in noise, for rapid speech, and for prolonged talking.

Esophageal Speech

Speaking with esophageal voice has been the goal of laryngectomees for half a century. Successful production of esophageal voice has been the yardstick by which rehabilitation was measured by the International Association of Laryngectomees (IAL). Certainly, more laryngectomees have attempted to use esophageal speech as the prime means of expressing language after total laryngectomy than by all other means combined. The fact is that only 50 to 70% of the laryngectomees succeed in acquiring functional esophageal speech. Because of its importance, a working knowledge of the basis and mechanism of esophageal voice is helpful to nurses.

See Gardner (1971), Diedrich and Youngstrom (1966), and Snidecor (1968) for details on esophageal speech.

On a mechanical level, speaking requires a source of power, a mechanism capable of being powered into vibration (tone), a tube to carry and amplify that tone, and a system of shaping a stream of air and tone into individual sounds for connected speech. For most people the lungs, larynx, vocal tract, and articulators serve the four functions. After the removal of the larynx by surgery, it is possible to replace the lung with the esophagus as an air storage tank. Further, the top of the esophagus has tissue, held under tension, which can be vibrated by air to produce sound. Fortunately, the esophagus, like the larynx, opens up into the bottom of the throat to carry tone produced.

The essence of speech with esophageal voice is to introduce air into the normally closed esophagus, to store it until needed, and to expel the air against the upper esophageal margins for tone.

Different techniques may be used to capture air into the esophagus. In essence, air may be drawn down or pushed down from the throat into the esophagus. Regardless of technique, entrance of air into the esophagus is made easier if that upper esophageal sphincter is reduced in tension. Once captured, air may be retained in the esophagus until pulsed up for speech. Once phonated, the sound may be carried through the throat and mouth to be resonated and articulated.

The nature of the esophagus as a substitute lung and pseudoglottis determines that esophageal tone is shorter in duration, lower in pitch, and softer in volume than voice from a larynx. The process also carries risks of taking too much time and effort to get air down, of having too audible an expulsion of lung air from the stoma when talking, and of failing to make speech consonants sufficiently precise. Within the limits and risks noted, esophageal speech can be developed to an intelligible degree for many laryngectomees.

Obstacles to learning range from reduced practice time, low motivation, and limited teaching opportunity, to physical factors such as significant hearing loss or other surgical treatment complications. Individuals who experience such problems may now be given another alternative form of oral communication: surgical techniques for postlaryngectomy voice rehabilitation.

Surgically Facilitated Voice

Contemporary history of surgical attempts to facilitate voice following laryngectomy is long and colorful. Numerous surgeons have described various procedures which focused on voice restoration after surgical removal of the larynx.

See Blom and Singer (1979) for an interesting account of the historical overview of surgery and associated prostheses to facilitate voice after laryngectomy.

Singer and Blom (1980) describe a simple puncture procedure and valved prosthesis for voice restoration for laryngectomees. The 30-minute surgical procedure, performed at any time following laryngectomy, involves creating a small fistula in the parting wall—the posterior wall of the trachea and the anterior wall of the esophagus. (See Figure 2–5.) A silicone valved prosthesis, termed a *duckbill* due to the similarity of the valved tip to a duck's bill is worn in the tracho-esophageal fistula to stent the tract and to prevent aspiration of food and saliva into the lungs.

The prosthesis, secured to the neck, extends from the patient's stoma to a point just inside the esophagus. When the stoma is occluded, or closed off with a finger, exhaled pulmonary air is shunted through the one-way, slit-like valve into the esophagus. Resulting esophageal voice has considerable duration.

The nurse can assist the patient by overseeing follow-up and reinforcing information taught to the patient/family by the surgeon/speech-language pathologist team. Learning proper placement and taping of the duckbill, as well as practice in speaking, are important aspects of the nursing care for these patients.

Recently, Panje (1981) has introduced a similar surgical procedure. A modified valved voice prosthesis, a *voice button*, is used to stent the tracheoesophageal fistula. The duckbill and the voice button devices have sparked a renewed drive to give improved tracheal-esophageal voice to laryngectomees. Both devices have met initial tests and acceptance.

FIGURE 2–5

The puncture technique for voice restoration after laryngectomy.

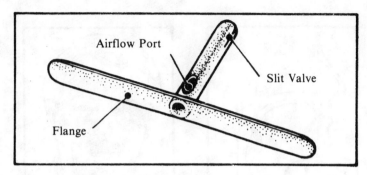

Airflow Port

Slit Valve

Flange

Voice Prosthesis

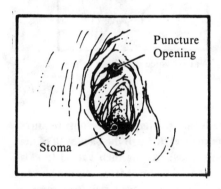

Puncture Opening

Stoma

1. Stoma and puncture opening for voice.

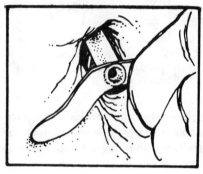

2. Voice prosthesis being inserted.

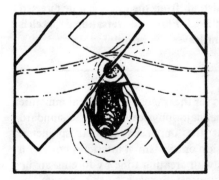

3. Voice prosthesis taped in place.

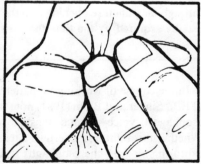

4. Blocking the stoma to direct air into the throat for voice.

FIGURE 2–5 (continued)

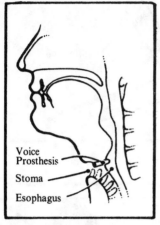

Voice prosthesis placement in "puncture" opening from stoma into throat

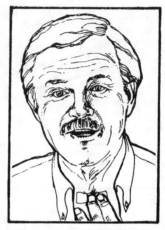

Valved voice prosthesis in place.

The "puncture" technique for voice restoration after laryngectomy requires a minor surgery to make an opening (puncture) through the back wall of the trachea (windpipe) into the throat (esophagus). A one inch valved tube is worn in the puncture opening at all times to prevent it from closing and to eliminate leakage during swallowing. It is removed once a day for cleaning.

The hospitalization requires 7–10 days during which time stoma care and voice training are provided. Voice is produced by blocking the stoma (breathing opening) with a finger so that exhaled air from the lungs can be directed through the puncture opening into the throat. Fluent conversational speech is usually acquired by the time the patient leaves the hospital.

In the course of working up patients for the tracheo-esophageal puncture (TEP), Singer and Blom (1981) note the major physical obstacle to standard esophageal voice—undue tension at the upper esophageal sphincter. Whether this tightness is termed a tension or a spasm, it interferes both with capturing air into the esophagus and with creating tone by forcing air up from the esophagus. An innovative surgical approach to this tension has been developed by Singer and Blom (1981). A myotomy interrupts the sphincteric integrity of muscles surrounding the top of the esophagus. Preliminary results are most promising. Indeed, history may judge this to be among the greatest contributions to providing voice, an essential feature of laryngectomee rehabilitation.

REFERENCES

Aronson, A.E. *Clinical voice disorders, An interdisciplinary approach.* New York: Thieme-Stratton, 1980.

Baker, B., & Cunningham, C. Vocal rehabilitation of the patient with a laryngectomy, *Oncology Nursing Forum*, 1980, 7, 23–36.

Batsakis, J. *Tumors of the head and neck:Clinical and pathological considerations.* Baltimore: Williams & Wilkins, 1974.

Blom, E., & Singer, M. Surgical-prosthetic approaches for postlaryngectomy voice restoration. In R. Keith & F. Darley (Eds.), *Laryngectomee rehabilitation.* San Diego: College-Hill Press, 1979.

Boone, D.R. *The voice and voice therapy.* Englewood Cliffs, NJ: Prentice-Hall, 1977.

Brodnitz, F.S. *Vocal rehabilitation.* Rochester, MN: Whiting Press, 1967.

Cooper, M. *Modern techniques of vocal rehabilitation.* Springfield, IL: C.C. Thomas, 1973.

Diedrich, W., & Youngstrom, K.A. *Alaryngeal speech.* Springfield, IL: C.C. Thomas, 1966.

Fisher, S. *Body experience in fantasy and behavior.* New York: Appleton-Century-Crofts, 1970.

Gardner, W.H. *Laryngectomee speech and rehabilitation.* Springfield, IL: C.C. Thomas, 1971.

Gonnella, C., Parker, D., Hollender, J., Lowell, G., Petterson, P., & Miller, S. *Normative criteria for cancer rehabilitation.* Atlanta, GA: Emory University, 1978.

Hannahs, K., Hooper, J., & Sigler, B. Nursing care of the head and neck cancer patient. In J. Suen & E. Myers (Eds.), *Cancer of the head and neck.* New York: Churchill Livingstone, 1981.

Lawson, W., & Biller, H. Cancer of the larynx. In J. Suen & E. Myers (Eds.), *Cancer of the head and neck.* New York: Churchill Livingston, 1981.

Lowry, W. Alcoholism in cancer of the head and neck. *Laryngoscope*, 1975, *85*, 1275.

Meyerson, M.D., & Shanks, S.J. Voice disorders in adulthood. In D.S. Beasley & G.A. Davis (Eds.), *Aging, communication processes and disorders.* New York: Grune & Stratton, 1981.

Moore, G.P. *Organic voice disorders.* Englewood Cliffs, NJ: Prentice-Hall, 1971.

Panje, W. Prosthetic vocal rehabilitation following laryngectomy—The voice button. *Annals of Otology, Rhinology, and Laryngology*, 1981, *90*, 116–120.

Singer, M., & Blom, E. A selective myotomy for voice rehabilitation after total laryngectomy. *Archives of Otolaryngology*, 1981, *107*, 670–673.

Singer, M., & Blom, E. An endoscopic technique for restoration of voice after laryngectomy. *Annals of Otology, Rhinology, and Laryngology*, 1980, *89*, 529–533.

Snidecor, J.C. *Speech rehabilitation of the laryngectomized.* Springfield, IL: C.C. Thomas, 1968.

Weinberg, E.G. *A child's cry—A clue to diagnosis.* New York: C. Pfizer, 1971. (Audio record)

Wilson, K. *Voice problems of children.* Baltimore: Williams & Wilkins, 1979.

Wynder, E. Toward the prevention of laryngeal cancer. *Laryngoscope, 1975, 85*, 1190.

Zemlin, W.R. *Speech and hearing science.* Englewood Cliffs, NJ: Prentice-Hall, 1968.

3

Hearing Impairment: Basic Information for Nurses

Dennis Arnst
George Purvis

HEARING IMPAIRMENT

Hearing impairment is an insidious problem which affects humans from conception throughout life. It takes many forms and relates to many causes, but the net influence is significant—it reduces communication ability. Hearing impairment often produces a form of isolation which has far-reaching effects on many people. Although the word *deafness* has been used to refer to partial as well as total hearing loss, the problems and needs confronting deaf persons and individuals with a partial hearing loss are quite different. The primary impact is determined by whether or not the hearing loss occurred before or after the acquisition of speech and language. Consequently, the onset of hearing loss is important to the remediation/rehabilitation process. To emphasize the difference, this Chapter contains information dealing strictly with *hearing impairment* and Chapter 4 will deal with the problem of *deafness*.

The purpose of this chapter is to provide the nurse with an overview of: (a) the procedures used for hearing assessment, (b) the types of hearing loss and resulting communication disorders, and (c) the hearing aid. References to readily available source material have been made so the reader can augment the information summarized here.

Onset of Hearing Loss

Development of the auditory system is a magnificent feat. The embryological precursors of hearing are first noted at 3 to 4 weeks of fetal development. During the 7th through the 12th week, the sensory part of the hearing mechanism—the cochlea—begins to unfurl. At the same time the structures of the middle ear are forming. By the 36th to 38th week, the entire ear system is functionally intact. Consequently, the auditory system is operational at birth—ready to receive and transmit sound to the auditory areas of the brain. But, any disturbance in this finely tuned process can result in poor auditory function, ranging from sensory deficits to reduced ability to process sound in the brain.

Even more remarkable than its development, is the ear's predisposition to deteriorate. The auditory mechanism is highly susceptible to many damaging influences. Disease processes, trauma, and environmental effects all play a role in reducing the effectiveness of the ear. In addition, aging undermines hearing by changing not only sensitivity to sound but also the ability to process information.

Children are affected by hearing impairments related to childhood disease or other trauma that occurs postnatally or that have roots in events which began during embryological development. Damaging influences on the auditory system are countless and often undermined. Compared to children, adults are confronted with an entirely different barrage of potential auditory problems, although incidence figures remain fairly constant. Otosclerosis, acoustic neuromas, and ototoxicity are auditory insults that generally afflict adults. The hearing of older persons is affected by the culmination of whatever influences occurred earlier in life as well as the effects of aging. Moreover, the automatic predisposition to hearing loss is hastened and complicated further by ever-present environmental noise. It should be evident that hearing impairment can occur throughout life from an endless number of causes.

Although the effects of hearing loss can often be devastating for those who experience them, the range of sensitivity loss and actual communication problems associated with hearing impairments differ widely. While hearing loss is part of natural aging, there are ways of dealing with the problem that can reduce the deleterious consequences. Although normal hearing can never be restored in most cases, communication can be facilitated with the use of a hearing aid. Unfortunately, the contact lens for the ear has not yet been realized. For the hearing impaired individual, the battle over a hard or soft prosthesis might be a welcomed confrontation, if only we could devise the Snellen Chart for hearing.

Prevalence of Hearing Loss

Incidence of hearing loss has been studied by many groups and in many ways. Data often vary due to the definition and classification system used to analyze results, along with other variables. But, it has been estimated that approximately 8.5 million persons in the United States have handicapping hearing loss in one or both ears. Northern and Downs (1978) reported that the average prevalence of hearing loss in children is about 10%, and, according to Gerber (1977), more than 1 in 1,000 newborns with hearing loss have been detected worldwide. A survey by the Office of Demographic Studies (1973) revealed that 700 out of 1,000 childhood hearing impairments were due to prenatal effects and 365 out of 1,000 were due to postnatal effects. Studies have indicated that the prevalence of hearing loss with advancing age was 52.2 per 1,000 for ages 45 to 64 and 129.9 per 1,000 for ages 65 to 74 (Maurer & Rupp, 1979). At present, approximately 10% of the total population of the United States is 65 years of age or older. It has been projected that by the year 2000, 17 to 18% of the population will have reached 65 years of age. This shift will, of course, shift the prevalence figures proportionately.

Impact of Hearing Loss

Current data indicate that there is a significant number of persons with hearing loss. However, the impact of the problem on each individual is not so neatly defined. Even with the use of hearing aids, communication difficulties persist but, based solely on the amount of deficit, are not totally predictable.

Since the primary impact of hearing impairment involves communication, early intervention/detection programs have been of concern for many years. The importance of establishing a communication system early has been emphasized for both hearing-impaired children and adults. Children whose hearing deficit occurs before their language has formalized experience a far greater handicap than those whose loss occurs after language has emerged. Much attention has been drawn recently to those children who suffer from chronic middle ear disorders. The potential effects of intermittent deprivation to language stimulation due to the hearing problem have been implicated in poor language processing abilities and learning deficits.

The primary impact of hearing loss in children relates to learning as well as communication. In adults, isolation and inability to follow established life patterns as hearing deteriorates creates the most significant problems. Young adults can adapt to the changes hearing loss brings with some assistance. Often the compensation occurs unnoticed. It is not until several rather abrupt communication confrontations that the results of the hearing deficit are felt. But the older adult who is undergoing an age-related isolation experience has greater difficulty dealing with hearing loss as it is an additional reminder of advancing age. The hearing deficit produces a "the-world-is-mumbling-so-why-bother" attitude and precipitates further removal from a once active life. Regardless of age, it is important to make sure each person with a hearing problem receives the best possible services.

Hearing Health Care Facilities

Programs to identify, assess, and rehabilitate hearing-impaired individuals can be located in many types of facilities. The primary hearing health care team involved in this process includes the otologist, the audiologist, and the hearing aid dispenser/hearing aid dealer. The otologist is responsible for the medical evaluation of the individual's hearing, while the audiologist provides the evaluation of hearing sensitivity and function. In addition, the audiologist usually coordinates habilitation/rehabilitation efforts directed toward alleviating the problems which accompany hearing loss. In cases of severe-to-profound hearing loss, specially trained personnel (e.g., educators of the deaf) figure significantly in the habilitation/rehabilitation plan. Should a hearing aid be advised, the team also includes the hearing aid dispenser/dealer who is responsible for fitting of the aid and related follow-up. In many cases, the audiologist is also certified as a dispenser and serves a dual function.

Identification programs are base-level sources of services for persons with hearing problems. Hearing identification efforts are focused in neonatal care units, public schools, industry, and well elderly clinics to locate those who may have auditory problems so that the rehabilitative process can be started. Hospitals and clinics—community, university, state, and federal—usually provide complete hearing health care services. Convalescent hospitals are required to provide audiologic services for the elderly. A permanent speech and hearing rehabilitation staff is usually not provided inhouse, but needed programs are available on a contractual basis with community facilities.

Although services for hearing impaired convalescent hospital patients can be obtained, a number of factors contribute to their under-utilization with this population.

(1) Most patients in convalescent hospitals are in an age group where hearing loss is very prevalent, most people involved (i.e., staff, physicians, family) feel nothing can be done to improve hearing anyway, so why bother.

(2) Older patients who have a hearing aid often have difficulty with care of the aid, insertion of the ear mold, and use of the aid in varying listening conditions due to physical limitations (e.g., arthritis, visual problems, manual dexterity).

(3) Often convalescent hospital staff lack awareness of procedures for obtaining needed audiologic assessment and aural rehabilitation management services.

(4) Added expenditures required to provide needed services, obtain hearing aids, and replace batteries often preclude consideration of seeking sources for those services.

In many cases inservice training sessions can be provided to familiarize all persons involved in the care of convalescent older patients with the problems of hearing loss and proper follow-up. The speech-language pathologist can be a ready source of information when an audiologist is not on staff.

Audiologists and otologists are found in private practice in separate as well as shared facilities. As the two professions work with the management of hearing impairment, this combination is natural. It should be remembered that the first step toward dealing with the needs of the hearing-impaired person is through medical examination of the ear and a complete test of the auditory system.

The Role of the Nurse

The nurse's role in the management of hearing impairment varies considerably and is often defined by the type of work facility. Nurses in acute care and convalescent hospitals and outpatient clinics deal peripherally with assessment and rehabilitation of hearing loss if the facilities do not have a speech and hearing program. If the setting has a program, the nurse's responsibilities are mainly to make sure patients who need help are referred for services, or to assist when a patient is having difficulty with a hearing aid.

In public schools the nurse assumes responsibility for coordinating the hearing screening program as directed by the state's department of health and or education. In most cases the nurse performs pure tone hearing screenings, maintains adequate health records, and serves as a source for related services. Hearing screening responsibilities may be incorporated into the job description for nurses employed in industry. Specific educational requirements, which vary from state to state, must be met to provide these services.

Nurses also carry out simple hearing screening procedures in offices of physicians in private practice. These tests, which are described in a later section, are basic and do not involve the extensive work-up provided by audiologists. In addition, the nurse may provide information to patients concerning related services.

Consequently, the nurse provides service as a facilitator and important source for information. Basic to that function is an understanding of the nature of hearing problems, their effects on people, related needs, and places where hearing impairment can be dealt with in an efficient manner. In some settings the nurse coordinates all related hearing health care services which will best benefit the patient.

MEANS OF DETECTING HEARING LOSS

Assessment of the auditory system involves tests designed to determine the sensitivity and functional abilities of the ear. Pure tone and speech materials are the basis of most evaluation procedures. Collectively, a battery of test results provides the best means of evaluating auditory problems. Screening programs usually provide entry level information concerning potential cases of hearing loss. No statement can be made regarding hearing status based on screening test results. The complete audiometric battery is the only way to determine a full picture of the patient's hearing problems.

Screening

One of the major goals of hearing screening programs is to identify individuals who have hearing impairments that interfere with or that have the potential to interfere with communication (Asha, 1975). Currently two methods of hearing screening are in use, pure tone and impedance audiometry.

Pure Tone Audiometric Screening

Traditionally, hearing screening programs have used pure tone air-conduction sensitivity tests as their basis. Attempts to utilize speech signals in screening programs have met with little success. Perhaps the most significant argument against the use of speech tests is the possibility that individuals with high frequency hearing loss will not be identified. While some attempts have been made to alleviate this criticism, speech screening is not widely used.

Perhaps the most popular hearing screening procedure over the years has been the constant intensity and limited frequency approach. In this procedure the intensity (loudness) dial of the audiometer is set at a constant level and tones are presented to a listener at a limited number of frequencies. The listener is asked to raise a hand, press a button or give a similar response each time a tone is heard. This type of procedure can be utilized with both adults and children. It must be emphasized that in this type of screening test we are not concerned with determining a threshold or lowest level at which a listener correctly identifies the presence of sound. The major emphasis is on the response to presence or absence of sound.

Since the goal of hearing screening is to identify individuals with actual or potential hearing impairments which will affect their communication, the selection of appropriate pass/fail criteria is critical. The intensity of a tone must not be so loud as to pass individuals with significant hearing loss or so soft that listeners with no hearing impairment will be failed. Likewise, the frequency range must not be so wide or restrictive that invalid test results are obtained. While many levels and test frequencies are proposed, Anderson (1978) suggests that it appears to be accepted today that one should use at least the frequencies 1000, 2000, and 4000 Hz (hertz—the unit of measurement of frequency) at levels no higher than 25 dB (decibel—the unit of measurement of loudness) (American National Standards Institute, 1969). The reader should be certain to check for any state or local requirements for level and frequencies to be utilized in a screening program.

The acoustic environment is an important variable in screening programs. While some screening programs may utilize sound-treated rooms, the vast majority are forced to operate in locations not entirely suitable for hearing testing. Usually these environments will be adequate for testing at frequencies above 1000 Hz, with occasional interference when screening at 1000 Hz. The potential for interference at 500 Hz is much greater than for higher frequencies. Caution must be exercised when using 500 Hz as a test frequency to ensure that the ambient noise levels are low enough as to not interfere with testing.

Careful placement of the earphones will decrease the loudness of environmental sounds. Do not, however, assume that the use of carefully fitted earphones replaces the need for a quiet testing environment.

When an individual fails to respond to a predetermined number of tonal presentations during screening, a referral for follow-up testing and or medical examination must be made. Wilson and Walton (1974) reported a 52% reduction in screening failures by rescreening. All failures should be rescreened preferably within the same session they failed, but definitely within one week after the initial screening failure (Asha, 1975). Rescreening is an essential procedure in improving the efficiency of a screening program.

Impedance Audiometry Screening

Pure tone air-conduction procedures are considered reasonably accurate in identifying individuals with hearing impairment. Melnick, Eagles, and Levine (1964), however, have shown that nearly one-half of the cases with active otologic pathology in their population were not identified using traditional screening techniques. The use of *impedance audiometry*, specifically tympanometry (a measurement of the mobility of the middle ear as a function of the differential pressure across the tympanic membrane) and acoustic reflexes (a stiffening of the middle ear as a result of the action of the stapedius muscle in response to a loud pure tone stimulus), has proven to be most helpful in identifying individuals with medical problems that might go unnoticed using traditional pure tone techniques. Advocates of impedance screening have specifically pointed to the failure of pure tone techniques in identifying individuals with mild losses due to middle ear disease. The potential danger of failing to identify mild losses caused by otitis media, is that even a mild hearing loss will cause unstressed words and less intense speech sounds (voiceless stops and fricatives such as p, t, k, s, f, th) to be inaudible, and this loss of auditory cues may create delays in normal acquisition of language (Skinner, 1978). The issue of mild hearing loss and delays in language acquisition is one of considerable discussion among speech-language pathologists. Nevertheless, it is an important consideration when advocating the use of impedance techniques in mass screening programs.

Numerous investigators have examined the use of impedance testing in mass screening programs. The widespread use of impedance screening has, however, not gained great popularity. McCandless (1979) has suggested that this is primarily due to the failure in establishing effective pass/fail criteria that can be employed with existing medical treatment and follow-up strategies. Bess (1980) has pointed out, that under one set of referral criterion, a child would be referred immediately upon failing the initial screening. Another set of referral guidelines recommends a retest in 4 to 6 weeks. It is possible that spontaneous recovery could occur in the 4- to 6-week time interval and no medical intervention would be necessary. Clearly one of the major issues in impedance screening is the potential for overreferral and overtreatment.

The questions surrounding impedance screening do not dispute its ability to identify middle ear pathology. It should be emphasized, however, that screening with tympanometry and the acoustic reflex is not a test of hearing. Significant sensorineural hearing loss may be present with normal impedance results. Conversely, abnormal impedance results can be observed in the presence of minimal hearing impairment. Utilizing a test battery (i.e., pure tone and impedance) is the most powerful approach to accurately identifying individuals with hearing impairment which interferes with communication.

Regardless of which procedure is used, the major emphasis of any screening program should be the early detection of hearing impairment. When an individual with hearing impairment is identified, further diagnostic tests, medical evaluation, and or treatment, and in some cases rehabilitation are in order. This more advanced testing should be done by an audiologist.

Complete Audiometric Testing

Screening tests are intended to identify problems for subsequent audiological and medical referral and are not diagnostic in the sense that they label specific disease entities. When an individual with a suspected hearing impairment has been referred for follow-up testing, the audiologist is basically interested in the severity of the hearing loss and what type of hearing disorder is present. When called on to answer these questions, the audiologist has at his or her disposal a number of tests to provide input into formulating a final diagnostic statement. Rosenberg (1978) has cautioned that no single test yields sufficient information to answer all diagnostic questions. While some tests will provide information primarily to assist in the determination of the existence of an auditory deficit, other tests will give information to specify the site of lesion. It becomes obvious that it is necessary to use an extensive battery of tests to ensure an accurate diagnosis of a hearing impairment.

The basic audiological test battery includes pure tone air conduction and bone conduction, speech reception thresholds, word discrimination testing, and the impedance test battery including tympanometry and acoustic reflex thresholds. This basic test battery will indicate if a conductive or sensorineural hearing impairment exists. In the event that no conductive component exists, further definition of the sensorineural hearing loss will be necessary to identify the specific site of lesion. Special tests which might be useful for this purpose include the Alternate Binaural Loudness Balance (ABLB) test, tone decay test, Short Increment Sensitivity Index (SISI), Bekesy Audiometry, acoustic reflex decay, and Performance Intensity (PI) function. While this is not an exhaustive list of tests available to the audiologist, it represents the major tests done to specify site of lesion in various types of sensorineural hearing impairments and found in a diagnostic report.

Test Equipment

In order to perform the basic audiological test battery, it is necessary to have an audiometer and impedance meter. The audiometer must have the capability of performing both pure tone and speech tests and should have two channels so that two independent signals may be generated and controlled separately. It should also have the ability to perform the special tests previously described. Whatever unit is used must meet certain standard requirements as stipulated by the American National Standards Institute (ANSI—1969). Such a unit is shown in Figure 3-1.

FIGURE 3-1

A clinical audiometer equipped to perform basic and advanced aduiometric tests (Courtesy of Maico Hearing Instruments, Inc.)

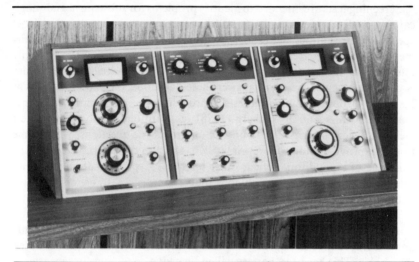

A portable audiometer may also be used in certain testing situations (Figure 3-2). Some portable units will only produce pure tone signals and will be used primarily in screening programs. Even though some units have the added capability of speech testing, the capability to perform many of the sophisticated site-of-lesion tests is limited.

An impedance meter is necessary for obtaining the tympanograms and acoustic reflex thresholds. A clinical impedance meter is shown in Figure 3-3, and a unit which might be used in a screening program is shown in Figure 3-4. Some units will not have the capability of producing a pure tone used to elicit an acoustic reflex. If this is the case, a separate pure tone audiometer will be necessary.

Test Environment

In order to obtain valid threshold measurements during the basic audiometric test battery, testing must be done in a relatively quiet setting. It is more crucial to control noise during threshold measurements, as opposed to screening programs, as we are interested in the softest tones a listener can perceive. Another important reason for controlling noise is that during pure tone bone conduction testing the ears are not covered by earphones.

FIGURE 3-2

A portable pure tone air conduction audiometer (Courtesy of Maico Hearing Instruments, Inc.)

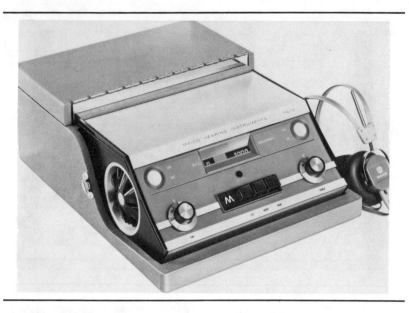

FIGURE 3-3

A clinical impedance meter used to perform tympanometry and acoustic reflex measurements (Courtesy of Grason-Stadler)

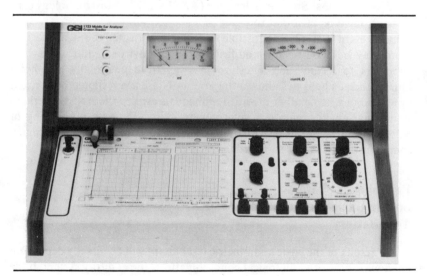

FIGURE 3–4

An automatic impedance meter used in hearing screening programs (Courtesy of Grason-Stadler)

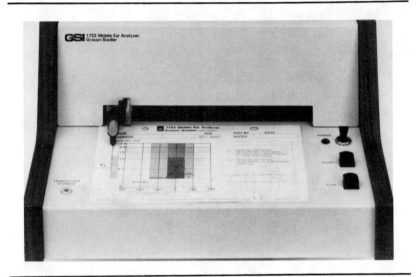

The most efficient means of controlling environmental noise during audiometric testing is by using a commercially manufactured prefabricated sound room (Figure 3–5). These rooms are manufactured to reduce noise to permissible levels at each of the audiometric test frequencies as specified by the American National Standards Institute (ANSI—1977). Most audiology clinics have this type of sound room.

In the event that it is not possible to use a prefabricated room, an existing room may be acoustically modified to reduce environmental noise. It is important to locate such a test room away from potentially high-noise sources such as hallways and waiting rooms. Noise levels should be checked by an audiologist or other qualified individuals against the ANSI criteria to assure that an adequate test environment exists. Periodic monitoring of noise levels should be done with both types of test rooms to ensure continued compliance with ANSI standards.

Pathological Effects on the Basic Audiometric Test Battery

The results of the basic audiometric test battery will be directly dependent upon what type of pathological condition affects the auditory system. If the

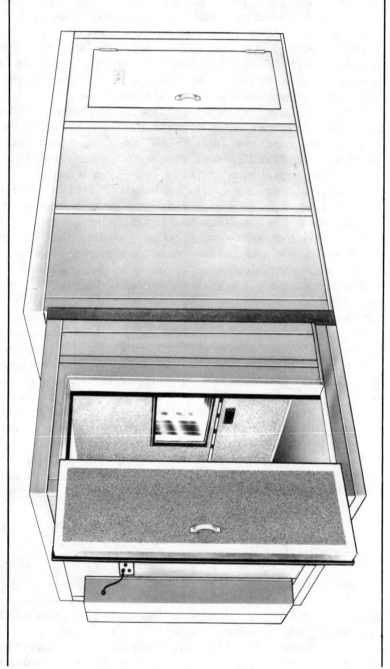

FIGURE 3-5 A two-room audiologic test suite suitable for basic and advanced audiologic testing (Courtesy of Industrial Acoustics Company, Inc.)

hearing loss is a result of any disorder of the pinna, external auditory meatus, tympanic membrane, or middle ear, abnormal test results will be observed on tests sensitive to the transmission of sound energy to the cochlea. This type of disorder is referred to as a *conductive hearing loss.*

When a hearing loss is a result of damage to the inner ear or cochlea, audiometric tests will show a reduction in sensitivity, in addition to the possibility of reduced ability to understand speech. This type of hearing loss is referred to as *cochlear* or *sensorineural hearing impairment.*

In the event damage occurs to the auditory portion of the VIIIth cranial nerve, the term *retrocochlear* is used. Some authors also include the low brain stem in this category. This type of hearing disorder may exist in the presence of normal hearing sensitivity but generally seems to be independent of and occurs across frequencies (Keith, 1980). There is a general trend in retrocochlear disorders, however, for a reduction in the ability to understand speech and also in the ability of the auditory system to maintain perception of a continuous pure tone over a brief period of time.

A *central hearing impairment* results from any disorder which influences the auditory pathways of the brain stem or the primary or association areas of the auditory cortex.. Auditory sensitivity in individuals with central hearing impairments will most always be normal. There will, however, in many instances be a breakdown in the ability to perceive speech in a complex listening situation, for example when two speech signals are competing. A more detailed discussion of each of the disorders described above will be covered in subsequent sections of this chapter.

Keith (1980) has stated that while the categorization of hearing impairment into distinct anatomical sites of conductive, sensorineural, and central impairment is convenient, it is seldom that simple in clinical practice. Multiple sites of lesions can and do exist and often present what appear to be conflicting test results. It is the challenging task of formulating a diagnostic statement by taking the results of the basic test battery and various special audiometric test procedures, that calls on the experience and training of the audiologist. The audiologist must examine the results of single tests and also obtain the feeling of the "gestalt" of the entire examination prior to making any statements regarding site of lesion (Rosenberg, 1978).

Audiometric Test Battery

Pure Tone Audiometry. A comparison of responses to pure tones presented (a) through the ear canal and (b) the bones of the head gives information as to the function of the middle ear. Individuals with normal middle ear function will show no difference in the thresholds measured by air conduction (with earphones on) and bone conduction (bone conduction vibrator placed on mastoid). When air conduction thresholds are worse than bone conduction thresholds, we say that an air-bone gap exists. This indicates that the middle ear function is abnormal, and is referred to as a *conductive disorder*.

Speech Audiometry. Two types of tests using speech stimuli are utilized during the basic audiometric test battery: (1) speech reception threshold (SRT) and (2) word discrimination tests.

One of the questions to be answered when evaluating a hearing impairment is the extent of the hearing loss. The SRT estimates the extent of the hearing loss for speech and tells us how loud speech must be in order for a listener to understand 50% of the speech material presented to him or her. This measurement is highly reliable and will agree very closely with an average of certain pure tone thresholds. The SRT also serves as a reference point from which to assess a listener's performance with speech materials presented at suprathreshold levels.

Word discrimination tests assess the ability of the listener to correctly perceive speech materials presented at levels above the threshold for speech. Since normal conversational speech does not occur at threshold, but at suprathreshold levels, word discrimination tests give a valid estimate of an individual's ability to understand everyday conversational speech. The ability to understand suprathreshold speech materials also serves as a diagnostic tool. Individuals with pure conductive losses will have normal word discrimination ability when the intensity of speech is sufficiently loud. Conversely, individuals with sensorineural pathology will generally show a reduction in the ability to understand speech as a function of the extent of cochlear damage.

Impedance Audiometry. Impedance audiometry has become an integral part of the audiometric test battery. Impedance measurements are particularly useful to audiologists because the objective results often substantiate or clarify behavioral results obtained by traditional audiometric tests. When interpreted properly, tympanometry and acoustic reflex tests yield useful information regarding middle ear function. It is often possible to determine subtle middle ear disorders when traditional air conduction and bone conduction tests are questionable. In addition to information regarding middle ear function, impedance measurements can also give diagnostic information relating to the cochlea, VIIIth nerve, and brain stem.

Special Audiometric Tests

Alternate Binaural Loudness Balance (ABLB). The ABLB test is the standard behavioral test of loudness recruitment. Recruitment is a phenomenon in which a relatively slight increase in the loudness of a sound results in a disproportionate increase in the sensation of loudness. Loudness recruitment is symptomatic of cochlear sensorineural hearing losses.

Tone Decay Test. Tone decay may be defined as the decrease in threshold sensitivity resulting from the presence of a continuous tone presented just above threshold or at suprathreshold levels. In this particular test, the listener is asked to indicate how long the presence of a tone is perceived. For individuals with conductive or cochlear hearing losses, there will be no difficulty in maintaining the perception of the tones for a brief period. Those with retrocochlear hearing impairments, however, will exhibit an inability to perceive a sustained tone.

Short Increment Sensitivity Index (SISI). The SISI is a test of a patient's ability to perceive a series of small 1 dB increments superimposed on a continuous pure tone presented at 20 dB above the threshold of the test frequency. The major contribution of this particular test is its ability to identify cochlear pathology. With newer and more accurate audiometric test procedures (e.g., acoustic reflex tests and brain stem audiometry), the SISI has become less used by the majority of clinical audiologists.

Bekesy Audiometry. Bekesy Audiometry is a testing procedure in which individuals trace their auditory thresholds on a self-recording audiometer. Jerger (1960) classified Bekesy test results by comparing the thresholds obtained with a continuous tone to those obtained with an interrupted tone. The four types of Bekesy audiograms proposed by Jerger give diagnostic information regarding site-of-lesion in the auditory system.

Acoustic Reflex Decay. The acoustic reflex is the contraction of the stapedius muscle in response to acoustic stimulation of high intensities. With continuous stimulation, the contraction of the stapedius muscle will be maintained until the stimulus ceases. The basis for the acoustic reflex decay test is that retrocochlear lesions produce a condition where the stapedius muscle cannot maintain contraction over a brief period of time. The ear with cochlear damage is characterized by its ability to maintain stapedial contraction for the duration of a sustained tonal stimulus.

Performance—Intensity Speech Discrimination Tests (PI). It is a recognized fact that as speech increases in intensity, it becomes more intelligible. A modification of speech testing procedures has been proposed by Jerger and Jerger (1971) to help identify retrocochlear pathology. Their procedure is based on the observation that as speech is increased in intensity, patients with cochlear impairment will reach a plateau and subsequent increases in intensity will have no effect on the speech intelligibility score. Individuals with retrocochlear pathology, however, will show a decrease in speech intelligibility as a function of increasing intensity. This phenomenon is called *rollover*.

The above list of special audiometric tests is not an exhaustive one. It does, however, represent the major tests one will encounter in reports of diagnostic audiological testing.

For basic information on audiology see:

F.N. Martin. *Introduction to Audiology*. Englewood Cliffs: Prentice-Hall, 1980.

D.E. Rose. *Audiologic Assessment*. Englewood Cliffs: Prentice-Hall, 1978.

J. Katz (Ed.). *Handbook of Clinical Audiology* (2nd ed.) New York: Williams & Wilkins, 1978.

S.E. Gerber and G.T. Mencher. *Auditory Dysfunction*. San Diego: College-Hill Press, 1980.

TYPES OF HEARING LOSS AND THE EFFECTS ON NORMAL AUDITORY FUNCTION

Normal hearing is something which has different meanings depending on the way in which the audiogram is viewed. The average person does not feel a hearing problem exists as long as there is no effect on social, vocational, or health status. The educator feels there is no hearing problem as long as there is no interference with educational progress. Some physicians limit hearing problems to those that cause health threatening conditions requiring medical intervention. All of these views make dealing with hearing disorders challenging and at times an exasperating experience.

Because there is no single means of defining the effects of hearing loss, all types of information must be taken into account. The first consideration is that of hearing sensitivity—How well does the ear respond to sound. Once this factor has been defined from a mechanical/physiological standpoint, the effects of that functional ability need to be related to the social, vocational, educational, and health aspects of the individual.

The remaining part of this section deals with: (1) a definition of normal hearing sensitivity, (2) a definition of hearing loss, (3) the functional effects of hearing loss on normal auditory function, and (4) general management foci for various types of hearing disorders. It will be assumed that the reader has a basic understanding of the anatomy of the ear.

For more information on anatomy and physiology, the reader is directed to the following source material:

J.D. Durrant and J.H. Lovrinic. *Bases of Hearing Science*. Baltimore: Williams & Wilkins, 1977.

S.E. Gerber. *Introductory Hearing Science: Physical and Psychological Concepts*. Philadelphia: W.B. Saunders, 1974.

V. Goodhill. *Ear: Diseases, Deafness, and Dizziness*. New York: Harper & Row, 1979.

W.R. Zemlin. *Speech and Hearing Science: Anatomy and Physiology*. Englewood Cliffs: Prentice-Hall, 1968.

FIGURE 3-6

Audiogram showing normal hearing bilaterally (right ear conduction = 0–0; left ear air conduction = X–X; right ear bone conduction = [–[; left ear bone conduction =]–])

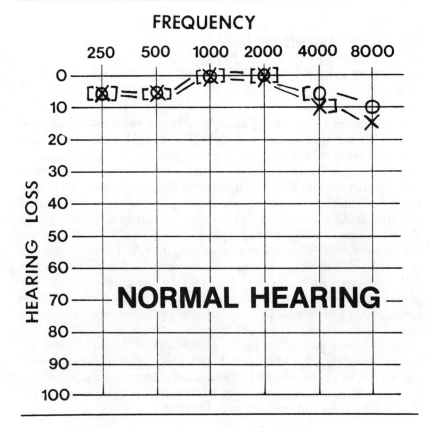

The Audiogram

All results from audiometric tests are reported on a special graph known as an *audiogram*. Figure 3–6 shows a sample audiogram commonly used by audiologists. The purpose of this graph is to report hearing test results systematically. The audiogram shown in Figure 3–6 shows the patient's hearing sensitivity. This information is plotted as a function of the frequencies (i.e., pure tones tested) and the intensity, or loudness. Space for various other tests are usually included on the audiogram form so the complete picture of the patient's auditory status can be evaluated. It is important to remember that the threshold of sensitivity represented on the audiogram reflects the softest sound the patient can hear. Any sound having a lower intensity will be inaudible to that patient.

Normal Hearing

Normal hearing occurs when sound is transmitted through the middle ear to the nerve endings in the cochlea and on through the auditory pathway to the brain centers without interruption or distortion. Normal hearing sensitivity is reflected on the audiogram with thresholds between 0–25 dB. All test results will fall within this range as is seen on the example audiogram in Figure 3–6. Functionally, no unusual behavior or test result will be noted. The exception will be the patient who is confused or annoyed because time was spent testing hearing in the first place. Others will display great relief to know "everything is fine."

Some difficulty may occur when the patient is convinced that a problem exists and that the tests cannot possibly reveal the true depth of the problem. In such cases, it is important that the patient be counseled that the full extent of hearing involves many aspects, including ability to attend to sound. Efforts are then focused on the fact that hearing is only one part of communication and that situational needs will vary that are under the control of the listener as well as the speaker.

Hearing Loss

Hearing loss is described in two ways (a) by amount of loss, and (b) by the type of loss. To determine the amount of hearing loss, the hearing sensitivity at 500, 1000, and 2000 Hz is averaged. The result is known as the *Three-Frequency Pure Tone Average* (PTA). Obviously, the greater amount of hearing loss, the greater the PTA and the patient's auditory problem. Categories have been established to quantify amount of hearing loss. These are:

Category	Hearing Loss Range
Normal	0–25 dB
Mild	26–40 dB
Moderate	41–70 dB
Severe	71–90 dB
Profound	90 dB or more

The relationship of these categories to the audiogram is shown in Figure 3–7.

FIGURE 3–7
Hearing loss categories plotted on an audiogram

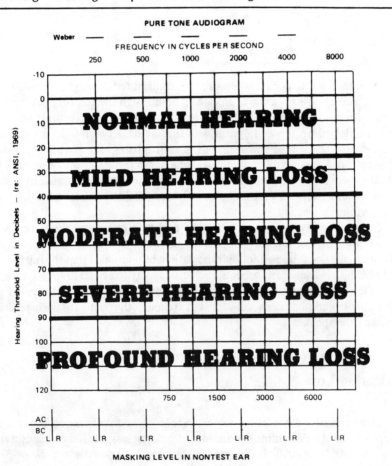

Specific hearing problems associated with each category vary and are influenced by the type of hearing loss. Also, sloping audiograms may be labeled with two categories (such as mild-to-moderate, moderate-to-severe, severe-to-profound) to reflect the change in severity of the hearing loss. The categories described here are a means to define the audiogram and should not be construed to imply explicit information about the hearing problems being experienced by the patient.

The type of hearing loss nomenclature relates to the physiologic problem precipitated by the pathology involved. The anatomy of the auditory system provides a convenient means of locating the area of dsyfunction. As can be seen in Table 3-1, there are four types of hearing loss which parallel the four major divisions of the auditory system. Although this anatomical-dysfunction paradigm is simple for educational purposes, in practice it makes the functional effects too discrete. The auditory system functions as a unit. The reader is cautioned against applying this as a hard-and-fast rule as many errors can be made and the real problem overlooked. Together, the amount and type of hearing loss provide a basic idea of the problems confronting the patient. The extent of testing will provide further information regarding the rehabilitative/habilitative needs and direction to be taken for each patient.

More information related to hearing loss can be found in the following references:

B.F. Jaffe. *Hearing Loss in Children.* Baltimore: University Park Press, 1977.

J.L. Northern. *Hearing Disorders.* Boston: Little, Brown and Company, 1976.

M.M. Paparella and D.A. Shumrick. *Otolaryngology* (Vol. 2). Philadelphia: W.B. Saunders, 1973.

H.F. Schuknecht. *Pathology of the Ear.* Cambridge, MA: Harvard University Press, 1974.

Conductive Hearing Loss

Conductive hearing losses affect the mechanical parts of the auditory system (i.e., the middle ear) and interfere with the delivery of sound to the nerve endings in the cochlea. No sound distortion is added to the auditory signal in this case. The primary problem in conductive hearing losses is the reduction in mechanical operation of the ear which reduces the loudness/intensity of the sound. Once the sound is made loud enough to exceed

TABLE 3–1

Summary of types of hearing loss and primary location of dysfunction

Type of Hearing Loss	*Location of Dysfunction*
Conductive	pinna—ear canal—middle ear
Sensorineural	Sensory: cochlea
	Neural: VIIIth nerve
Retrocochlear	VIIIth nerve—Low brain stem
Central	High brain stem—auditory cortex

the effects of the conductive problem, the patient can usually understand speech easily (providing no other problem exists). This makes the person with a conductive type of auditory disorder a prime candidate for a hearing aid. Medical remediation possibilities must be exhausted before the aid is considered, as a conductive hearing loss is often amenable to medical intervention (i.e., medication and or surgery).

Audiometric results. An example audiogram reflecting a conductive hearing loss is shown in Figure 3–8. Note the reduced air conduction thresholds (0–0s) reflecting the mechanical problem in the middle ear and the good bone conduction thresholds ([-[). The separation between the two results is known as an *air-bone gap* and is the hallmark of a conductive-type hearing loss. The size of the air-bone gap does not relate directly to specific factors. However, whenever the middle ear function is impeded, an air-bone gap will be reflected on the audiogram. Impedance audiometry is extremely important in identifying these types of problems as it is based on a measure of the mechanical aspects of the auditory mechanism.

It is possible that the effects on the middle ear mechanism reduce sensitivity to the limits of normal hearing (i.e., 25 dB-HL) and an air-bone gap occurs within this range (see Figure 3–9). This problem will produce minor effects on loudness transmission of sound to the cochlea, and if it occurs for a relatively short period of time (e.g., 4 to 6 weeks) and is temporary, no long-range effects will be noted. However, when an air-bone gap occurs and is related to a chronic problem, the reduction in hearing sensitivity can become a more substantial problem. Recently, attention has focused on the possibility of chronic conductive hearing loss (i.e., chronic otitis media) in children (ages birth to 5 years) creating a sound deprivation condition that affects speech and language development. The effects implicated in such cases relate to central aspects of hearing—those that involve the brain processes necessary for interpreting the sounds used in communication and

FIGURE 3–8

Example audiogram showing a conductive hearing loss for the right ear (air conduction = 0–0; bone conduction = [–[)

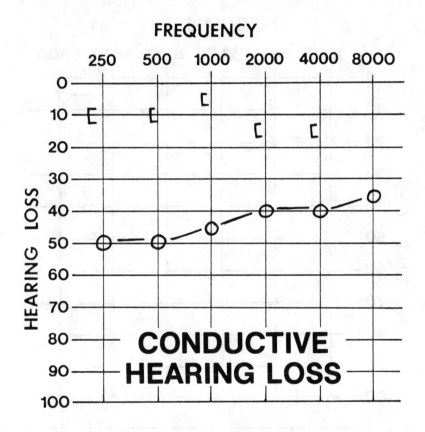

language learning. More work is being carried out to better define these effects on children who suffer from chronic middle ear problems.

The point to be stressed is that hearing screening programs may miss minimal conductive hearing losses and pass patients as hearing normally when, in fact, a minimal disturbance is present. The extent of this false-positive finding needs to be more carefully evaluated. But caution should also be exerted when nurses are receiving conflicting reports from others indicating a hearing problem appears to exist when the hearing screening results suggest a "pass."

FIGURE 3-9

Example audiogram showing a conductive hearing loss for the left ear with thresholds at the limits of normal hearing (air conduction = X–X; bone conduction =]–])

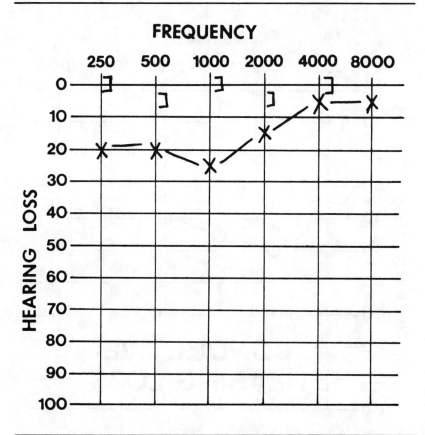

Causes. Causes for conductive hearing loss are summarized in Table 3–2. Although this is not an exhaustive list, the effect of all these problems involves delivery of the sound to the cochlea.

Management focus. The primary focus for management in cases of conductive hearing loss is medical intervention. Medication to treat middle ear effusion or removal of debris in the ear canal usually relieves the problem. In other cases, surgical intervention may be necessary, ranging from a simple procedure (e.g., placement of ventilating tubes) to a more complicated procedure (e.g., replacement of the stapes with a prosthesis in otosclerosis or

TABLE 3–2

Selected causes of conductive type hearing disorders

Congenital malformation of the middle ear mechanism
Perforation of the tympanic membrane
Fluid/infection in the middle ear (e.g., otitis media)
Objects lodged in the ear canal (e.g., cerumen, beans, erasers)
Fixation of the middle ear mechanism
Disruption of the middle ear mechanism (e.g., cholesteotoma)
Scar tissue on the ear drum (e.g., tympanosclerosis)
Poor Eustachian tube function

---

rebuilding the ear canal or pinna in atresia). When medical intervention has been exhausted, is contraindicated, or has been unsuccessful, hearing aids are the secondary approach to remediation of the problem. Amplification in cases of conductive hearing loss is usually very successful.

Sensorineural Hearing Loss

Cochlear (sensorineural) hearing losses affect the nerve endings and the ability to transmit sound through the central auditory pathway to the brain for processing. The effect of cochlear hearing loss is to introduce distortion and reduce intelligibility of speech sounds. Unlike conductive hearing losses, making the sound louder will not compensate completely for the auditory problem. In fact, most patients with cochlear hearing losses tend to have an abnormal sensitivity to loudness known as *recruitment*. This factor often limits the use of amplification but does not rule it out. Today's technology has brought the use of the hearing aid into the rehabilitation realm for patients with cochlear hearing disorders.

Audiometric results. A typical audiogram found in cases of cochlear hearing loss is shown in Figure 3–10. Note the reduced thresholds, particularly in the high frequencies. This type of pattern characterizes cochlear hearing problems. No air-bone gap is found in these cases as the middle ear mechanism is unaffected. Only the cochlea has been damaged. Cochlear hearing losses are also known as *sensorineural* losses as the sensory aspects of the ear—the nerve endings in the cochlea—are malfunctioning and the nerve or neural part of the system may also be involved beyond the cochlea.

FIGURE 3–10

Example audiogram showing sensorineural hearing loss for the right ear (air conduction = 0–0; bone conduction = [–[)

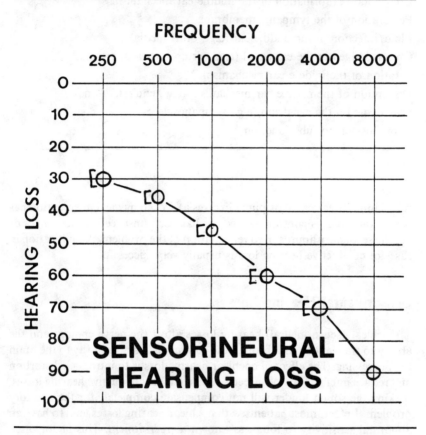

Occasionally, thresholds are poorer in the low frequencies than in the highs. This type of audiometric configuration is associated with Meniere's disease, the effects of aging, or brain stem disorders. In all cases, site of lesion testing is necessary to help differentiate the exact problem being reflected on the audiogram.

One major effect of the distortion produced by cochlear type hearing problems is reflected in poor *Word Discrimination Scores* (WDS). The nerve endings are incapable of coding enough information for the brain to interpret the sound going into the ear adequately. A similar result can be obtained when a stereo system has a faulty speaker or the radio has not been precisely tuned to a station. Information required to understand the sounds being transmitted is often reduced.

TABLE 3-3

Selected causes of sensorineural hearing loss

Congenital malformation of the cochlea

Viral infections (e.g., mumps)

Head injury/trauma

Meningitis

Meniere's disease

Ototoxicity

Noise exposure (prolonged)

Demyelinating diseases (e.g., multiple sclerosis)

Genetic influences/syndromes

Aging

Causes. Sensorineural hearing loss is caused by a wide variety of sources; these are summarized in Table 3-3.

In some cases, patients with cochlear problems also experience middle ear problems. This combination effect adds the influences of a conductive hearing loss to those related to the sensorineural problem. An example of this *mixed type hearing loss* is shown in Figure 3-11. Note the decreased bone conduction thresholds which reflect the condition of the cochlea, and the air-bone gap which indicates the mechanical problem affecting the middle ear.

Management focus. Medical intervention in cases with cochlear hearing loss is not possible. No treatment or surgical intervention can replace damaged transmission properties of the cochlea. Approaches such as cochlear implants and modification of congenital or hereditary aspects of sensorineural hearing loss are presently being persued but remain experimental and speculative. Surgery to alleviate the vertiginous attacks associated with Meniere's disease is considered only in selected individuals, but not as a corrective procedure for loss of hearing.

Aural rehabilitation/habilitation is the primary management approach for sensorineural hearing loss cases. It is directed at dealing with the very real problems facing poor transmission in the ear. When indicated, amplification is most useful to assess this process; however, the hearing aid can only make sounds *louder* not *clearer*. Due to this limitation, restoration of hearing to *normal* function is not possible. The hearing aid wearer must come to understand and accept this principle, and deal with communication situations as best as possible. When hearing has been damaged from birth, it is

FIGURE 3–11

Example audiogram showing a mixed type hearing loss for the left ear
(air conduction = X–X; bone conduction =]–])

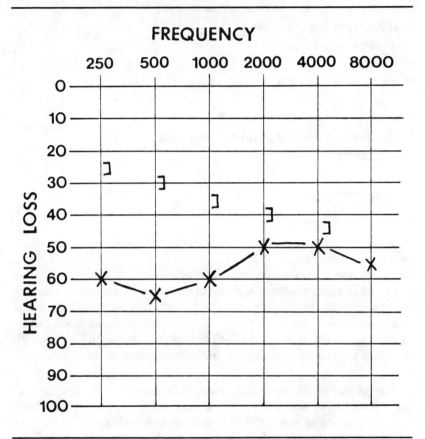

important to consider the use of amplification very early along with some
means of communication. In most cases manual signs and the manual
alphabet should be considered to facilitate development of language skills. It
is extremely important that children with severe hearing loss be provided a
means to interact with the world around them. Without that interaction, the
possibility of language and communication is severely limited.

Retrocochlear Hearing Loss

Retrocochlear hearing loss is generally confined to problems affecting the
VIIIth cranial (auditory) nerve and the low brain stem area. This type of

hearing problem is not very common in children and is usually due to a tumor or some other disease process or trauma which affects the transmission properties of the nerve to the brain. In most cases the patient reports a sudden onset of hearing loss in one ear accompanied by various other symptoms such as tinnitus (i.e., ringing in the ear) and or dizziness.

Audiometric results. Retrocochlear hearing loss does not produce typical findings on the audiogram. An example audiogram is shown in Figure 3–12.

FIGURE 3–12
Example audiogram showing a retrocochlear hearing problem (right air conduction = O–O; left air conduction = X–X; right bone conduction = [–[; left bone conduction =]–])

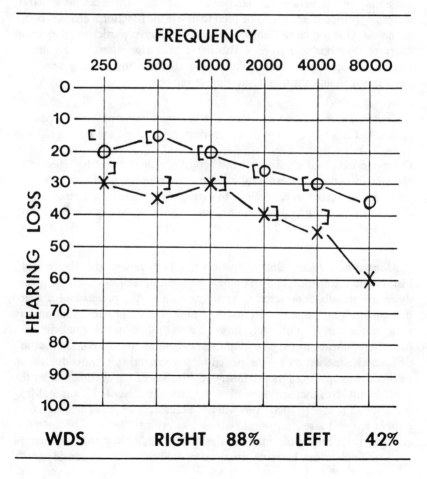

The most significant indicator is the unilateral sensorineural hearing loss and the unusually poor WDS in that ear. In some cases, the hearing loss is so minimal that pure tone thresholds are not shifted significantly. The hallmark sign is a WDS which appears to be inconsistent with the audiogram—minimal hearing loss with reduced WDS. Additionally, the acoustic reflex thresholds (ART) cannot be elicited. In cases not involving the VIIIth nerve, with the same amount of hearing loss, the ART would be present. Consequently, speech audiometry and impedance audiometry are extremely important tests to use when dealing with a suspected retrocochlear case. These diagnostic flags would suggest further verification with objective procedures such as *Auditory Brain Stem Response* (ABR) audiometry. (ABR is an electrophysiological means of evaluating the response of the auditory system.) Expanded speech audiometry procedures would also be employed to evaluate effects of the disorder on the transmission of speech. In particular, the ability of the patient to understand words and sentences presented at increasingly loud levels would be used to assess the functional characteristics of the ear. One speech audiometry procedure which is particularly helpful in differentiating cochlear from VIIIth nerve problems shows poorer understanding of speech at louder intensity levels than any other group. This pattern is a significant diagnostic sign in retrocochlear cases.

Causes. Retrocochlear disorders are the least common type of hearing problem. Causes for this type of hearing impairment are summarized in Table 3–4.
Often the increased invasion of the acoustic neuroma will be reflected in changes in audiologic test results. At present some procedures have been devised which claim to be sensitive to extremely small lesions. Retrocochlear disorders are not often detected until they have reached fairly large proportions, and have decreased function of the auditory nerve significantly.

Management focus. Once suspicion has been raised with the patient's history and the medical and audiologic evaluation, various radiologic procedures are usually considered to verify and locate the presence of a space occupying lesion. If confirmation can be obtained, surgical intervention may then be considered. Following surgery, aural rehabilitation (including the use of amplification) may be employed depending on the communication difficulties experienced by the patient. As a general rule, individuals with retrocochlear hearing loss are not good candidates for hearing aids as the problem involves the transduction of the nerve impulses to the brain. Making a sound louder in such cases will not necessarily improve hearing. If the patient has had a sensorineural hearing loss prior to the onset of the retrocochlear problem, an aid may be considered. Counseling and information for handling various listening situations would definitely be considered.

TABLE 3-4

Selected causes of retrocochlear hearing disorders

Meningioma, or schwannoma
Lymphoma
Glomus jugulare tumors
Neurofibroma
Pontine glioma

Central Auditory Disorders

Central auditory dysfunction cannot be considered a hearing loss as the problem relates to the processing of information in the auditory pathway and brain. The disorder in this case often reflects an inability to interpret the auditory signal transmitted through an intact middle ear and cochlea. The problem is more like a short circuit in a radio than the poorly tuned signal that results in cochlear disorders. In many ways, this type of auditory problem is the most difficult to deal with simply because it is as yet the least well understood. Moreover, it is often passed over as medical remediation is not possible and identification tools are just beginning to emerge. Also, test results cannot be categorized neatly as processing in the central nervous system is very complex.

Audiometric results. There is no example audiogram which can be ascribed to a central auditory problem. It has been known for quite some time that pure tones are unaffected by lesions in the central auditory pathway. Therefore, little effect is noticed on the audiogram. Speech audiometry, however, has been used to assess the problem by reducing the amount of information available in the speech signal. Special tests have been devised which add competing messages, filter part of the material, or present different speech materials to both ears at the same time. The distorted information can be analyzed by an unaffected central auditory system, but cannot be organized by the disordered auditory pathway.

Often inconsistencies in test results and behavioral data are the only clues to the problem. Yet, it is unwise to label the problem as "central auditory dysfunction" in an effort to call the problem something. Careful evaluation of behaviors noted and test results is extremely important. Input from the speech-language pathologist is often helpful. As the auditory problem relates to the organization and interpretation of speech and language signals, the entire communication system of the individual is affected.

Causes. A wide variety of problems can cause or be labeled as central auditory dysfunction—sometimes appropriately and sometimes inappropriately. Most obvious are the aphasias or other neurologic disorders that are clearly the result of an identifiable event in the patient's history (e.g., stroke, head trauma). On the other hand, processing difficulties have also been related to learning disabilities in children—problems not related to space-occupying lesions. Functional interaction of the various aspects of the auditory system are many and extremely interconnected. Total function of the processing system required for speech and language involves much of the brain. At present, efforts are being directed toward increasing the ability to identify and subsequently remediate the problem.

Management focus. Unless the central auditory problem is directly caused by stroke, head trauma, or other brain lesions, medical intervention is impossible. Medical clearance is necessary to be sure that lesions have been controlled or eliminated as possible causal factors. Once it has been obtained, aural rehabilitation and speech/language intervention remain the primary courses of action. In the case of aphasia, retraining auditory comprehension is incorporated into the work of the speech-language pathologist. Learning disabled children with central auditory disorders should also be referred to the speech-language pathologist for special training. In all cases of central auditory dysfunction, the use of amplification is contraindicated unless a physically definable hearing loss can be determined. Sending a louder signal through a system with a coding problem will not solve the needs of the individual.

A note of caution. Older adults not only have significant cochlear hearing problems, but also experience age-related processing problems. In many cases the resulting behavior places the patient in a category of "confused and disoriented." Unfortunately, the implied condition tagged to this label is *senile dementia.* Auditory problems can confuse older individuals and leave them disoriented. Consequently, more careful attention needs to be drawn to the specific conditions of senility. Hearing status should be evaluated carefully before notes or other statements relating or suggesting senility are entered into charts or other records of older adults.

Behavioral Indices

Conductive and sensorineural hearing impairments often manifest themselves in observable behavioral symptoms. While the symptoms cannot be used independently for diagnosis, they can be used as guides for further referral.

Individuals who exhibit conductive hearing impairments are often observed to speak in a quiet voice. This occurs even in the presence of high levels of environmental noise where a person with normal hearing typically raises the level of the voice. This may occur because the loss of sensitivity associated with the conductive disorders creates a condition in which the speaker is unaware of the extent to which environmental noise is interfering with his or her speech, and consequently does not realize the need to speak more loudly (Giolas, 1977). Another hypothesis is because the cochlea is intact, the individual hears through bone conduction and thus has no cue to speak louder.

Individuals with conductive hearing impairment often report that they hear better is the presence of noise, a symptom known as *paracusus willisiana*. Also observed in cases of middle ear disorders is an increased tolerance for sounds of high intensity due to the attenuation caused by the hearing impairment.

Sensorineural hearing impairment presents behavioral symptoms which are often in opposition to those seen in conductive losses. For example, the individual with a sensorineural disorder tends to speak louder than is appropriate for a particular situation. Unlike the person with a conductive disorder, the individual cannot take advantage of hearing through bone conduction and must speak louder.

Speech discrimination ability in an individual with sensorineural loss will typically be reduced regardless of the intensity of the speech signal. It is not uncommon to hear a person with this type of loss say, "I can hear, but I can't understand." Speaking louder will not necessarily help an individual with sensorineural impairment, but slowing down, enunciating clearly, and repeating statements are recommended methods of assisting this patient. Moreover, presence of background noise is most always reported as creating a more difficult listening situation for the person with sensorineural loss.

Sensorineural hearing losses generally cause an abnormal reaction to increases in loudness. If so, a signal will be perceived as being comfortable at one intensity, but with even a slight increase of intensity, the signal will be perceived as much too loud. This phenomenon, referred to as recruitment, can create significant problems for a person with a sensorineural hearing impairment who needs to wear a hearing aid.

Tinnitus, ringing in the ear or head noise, is a symptom of both conductive and sensorineural hearing impairments. When an individual notices a sudden onset of tinnitus or an increase in the intensity of tinnitus, referral for a medical and audiological evaluation is recommended. While tinnitus is not a disease itself, it is a signal that some type of hearing impairment is present.

HEARING AIDS

For those individuals who cannot benefit from medical treatment of their hearing impairment, a hearing aid may be recommended as a means of

FIGURE 3-13

Basic components of a hearing aid (From: W. Staab. *Hearing Aid Handbook.* Blue Ridge Summit: Tab Books, Inc., 1978. Reprinted by permission)

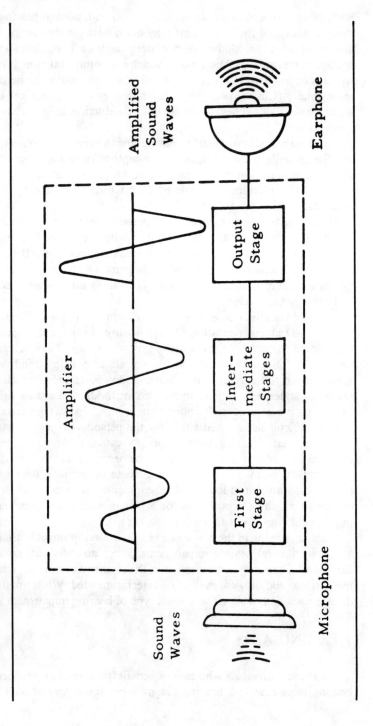

alleviating their communication problems. Hearing aids may, or may not, however, provide the expected help. In many instances a basic understanding of how a hearing aid functions and the benefits to be expected from wearing an aid can help in the successful adjustment to the aid.

A hearing aid is basically a device which makes sound louder. Early attempts by mankind to aid hearing were probably achieved by cupping the hands behind the ear. This not only served the purpose of collecting sound energy and directing it to the ear, but also alerted those around the hearing impaired individual to speak louder. From this rather crude beginning we have progressed to the modern electronic hearing aids of today.

Hearing Aid Components

Hearing aids are complex electronic devices. Despite the complexity of the internal circuitry, however, four basic components of a hearing aid can be identified (Figure 3–13): Microphone, amplifier, receiver, and power supply (battery).

The microphone collects sound energy and converts that energy into a weak electronic current.

The amplifier receives the weak electronic signal generated by the microphone and increases the amplitude (i.e., makes the signal louder). The amount of increase will be proportional to the number of stages in the circuit. Generally, the more stages (transistors and associated circuitry) the greater or louder will be the amplification.

The receiver is basically a miniature speaker. This component converts the amplified electrical signal into sound energy similar to that initially received by the microphone. It is this amplified signal which is then directed into the ear of the hearing impaired individual.

The battery is necessary to provide power to the amplifier. A battery in a modern hearing aid will last approximately 2 weeks. This will vary, however, with more powerful hearing aids using batteries more rapidly.

When the sound leaves the receiver it is necessary to provide a means of directing the signal into the ear canal. This is accomplished by use of a custom-fitted ear mold. Ear molds are made by taking an impression of the outer ear and sending the impression to a laboratory that will produce a finished mold. If the sound escapes from the ear canal and is picked up by the microphone, it will be further amplified. When this occurs a high pitch "squeal" will be heard. This sound is referred to as *feedback*.

Types of Hearing Aids

Hearing aids generally fall into two categories: *body and ear-level aids*. The body hearing aid (Figure 3–14) is generally worn on the chest, either in a shirt

FIGURE 3–14

Conventional body-type hearing aid (From: W. Staab. *Hearing Aid Handbook.* Blue Ridge Summit: Tab Books, Inc., 1978. Reprinted by permission)

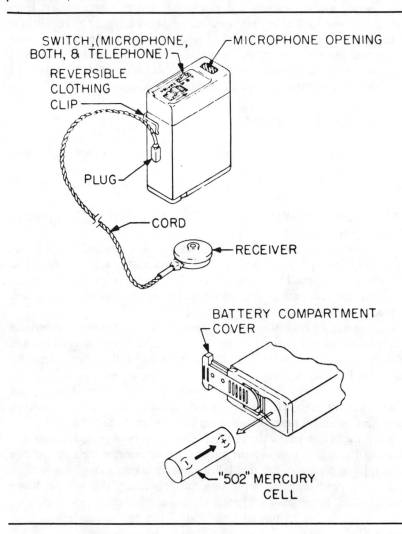

SWITCH,(MICROPHONE, BOTH, & TELEPHONE)

MICROPHONE OPENING

REVERSIBLE CLOTHING CLIP

PLUG

CORD

RECEIVER

BATTERY COMPARTMENT COVER

"502" MERCURY CELL

or coat pocket or in a harness made specifically for the hearing aid. The microphone, amplifier, and battery are contained within the case of the hearing aid. A cord carries the electrical signal to the receiver which is attached to the ear mold placed in the external ear. This type of hearing aid is

FIGURE 3–15

Behind-the-ear hearing aid (From: W. Staab. *Hearing Aid Handbook.* Blue Ridge Summit: Tab Books, Inc., 1978. Reprinted by permission)

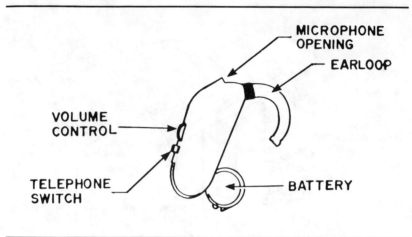

generally worn by children and adults with profound hearing losses. Occasionally individuals with arthritis or other problems which might interfere with manipulation of the smaller controls of the ear-level aid will be fitted with a body aid. The body aid typically has more accessible controls and is easier to operate for those with impaired movement.

Most individuals prefer to wear smaller ear-level hearing aids. In virtually all ear-level aids the four basic components are housed in a single plastic case, either behind-the-ear or in a mold which fits in the ear canal.

The behind-the-ear hearing aid (Figure 3–15) hangs behind the ear and has an earloop which attaches to a polyethylene tube coming from the ear mold. This is the most common type of hearing aid worn today. Because of recent advances in the field of electronics, this hearing aid can fit virtually all types and degrees of hearing loss.

If a patient wears glasses, a hearing aid built into the frame may be preferred (Figure 3–16). Although this type of hearing aid is preferred by some patients for cosmetic reasons, it has several disadvantages. The eyeglass hearing aid is not satisfactory if the patient uses glasses on a parttime basis or requires two or more different kinds of glasses. It is also not practical for the patient who requires parttime use of the hearing aid. A patient who requires frequent lens changes (e.g. cataract patients) will also find this type of hearing aid unsatisfactory (Hartford, 1979).

FIGURE 3–16

Eyeglass-type hearing aid (From: W. Staab. *Hearing Aid Handbook.* Blue Ridge Summit: Tab Books, Inc., 1978. Reprinted by permission)

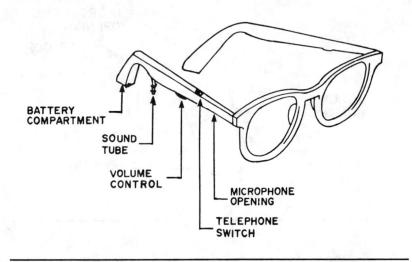

BATTERY
COMPARTMENT

SOUND
TUBE

VOLUME
CONTROL

MICROPHONE
OPENING

TELEPHONE
SWITCH

FIGURE 3–17

An in-the-ear hearing aid (From: W. Staab. *Hearing Aid Handbook.* Blue Ridge Summit: Tab Books, Inc., 1978. Reprinted by permission)

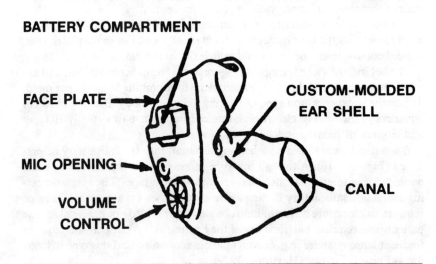

BATTERY COMPARTMENT

FACE PLATE

CUSTOM-MOLDED
EAR SHELL

MIC OPENING

VOLUME
CONTROL

CANAL

Recently, *in-the-ear* hearing aids (Figure 3–17) have gained popularity. This is due to the cosmetic appeal of this type of hearing aid. Many individuals feel that by using this type of aid they can hide their hearing impairment. Because of the great cosmetic appeal of this type of aid, some individuals have been fitted at their insistance while their hearing loss is too severe to benefit from an in-the-ear aid.

Hearing Aid Problems

It is beyond the scope of this chapter to make the reader an expert in the detection and troubleshooting of malfunctioning hearing aids. There are, however, several things that may be checked before sending the patient with a defective hearing aid to the audiologist.

If there is no sound coming through the aid, first check the battery to be sure that it is inserted properly and that the compartment is closed tightly. The battery case will have a small "+" sign which *must* be matched with the identical marking on the battery. If the hearing aid still produces no sound, insert a fresh battery. While this will be adequate in most instances, be aware that the new battery you assume is fresh may also be dead. Ideally, every battery should be checked with a voltage tester to assure that it possesses adequate current.

If the battery is functional and the hearing aid still does not produce any sound, check the ear mold. The ear mold will contain a small opening through which the sound from the hearing aid will be transmitted into the ear canal. If for any reason this opening becomes obstructed (e.g. blocked with ear wax), no sound will be heard from the hearing aid. If a blockage is observed, it may sometimes be removed by a toothpick, pipe cleaner, or paper clip that has been straightened out. The hearing aid and ear mold should be sent to an audiologist if these techniques are unsuccessful in removing any blockage. *Never attempt to remove wax from any opening of an in-the-ear hearing aid.* You may damage the microphone and or receiver. Also check to see that the tubing connecting the earloop of the behind-the-ear aid to the ear mold is not twisted or plugged with moisture.

Another problem, especially with new hearing aid users, is a lack of familiarity with the aid controls. Be certain that the hearing aid is turned on and the volume is turned up. Some hearing aids will have the on-off switch built into the volume control wheel. In this case as you increase the volume, the hearing aid will be turned on. Other models, however, have a separate on-off switch. Be certain that this switch is in the *on* position. Some aids will have a microphone-telephone switch. If the switch is in the T (telephone) position, the aid will be set to function with the magnetic signal from the hand piece of a telephone serving as the input signal instead of an acoustic signal. When this occurs many individuals mistakenly assume that the aid is not functioning properly because they do not hear any environmental sounds.

If the hearing aid does not function after checking the above items, send it to an audiologist. Remember a hearing aid is an extremely delicate instrument. Do not try to fix it yourself!

Occasionally feedback may become a problem for the individual wearing a hearing aid and or those around him or her. When feedback occurs it is sometimes the result of an improperly fitted mold, cracked tubing, or internal damage to the receiver. If the ear mold is not properly inserted, make any necessary adjustment. If feedback persists after proper insertion of the mold, refer the hearing aid user to an audiologist. If the ear mold makes the ear of the user sore, send the patient immediately to an audiologist for adjustment.

Many problems which affect hearing aids can be avoided if the aid is handled with care and a few simple precautions followed.

1. Never expose the hearing aid to excessive heat. Avoid placing the aid on a hot radiator or in the glove compartment of a car.
2. Do not allow the hearing aid to become wet. Remove the aid before showering or swimming. Should the hearing aid become wet, immediate action may preserve it if the following steps are followed:

    a. Remove the batteries at once.
    b. Wipe the exterior of the case with a dry absorbent cloth.
    c. Place the aid in a warm place. It is possible to use the low heat setting of a hair dryer. *Never place an aid in an oven.*

3. Never take the hearing aid apart to examine the insides. Guarantees may be made void by such action.

4. Never use alcohol, acetone, or cleaning fluid on a hearing aid. Wipe the case with an absorbent cloth, if necessary.
5. Do not wash the ear mold in alcohol, acetone, cleaning fluid, or extremely hot water. Chemicals may dissolve the plastic material of the ear mold. Hot water may soften the plastic and allow the ear mold to change shape.
6. If excessive dirt or wax collect on the mold, wash it in warm water using a mild soap. *Remove the mold from the hearing aid prior to washing.* Wipe excess water from the mold, blow to clear any moisture from the tube, and allow the aid to dry overnight.
7. Discard any batteries which appear to be leaking at once. Clean the battery case immediately.

8. Remove the hearing aid at night and place out of reach of small children and pets.
9. Remove batteries or open the battery case when the aid is not in use. Some aids will continue to drain current from the battery even with the volume turned down.

Misconceptions and Limitations of Hearing Aids

A popular misconception held by many is that once a hearing aid is fitted to an individual with a hearing impairment, the ability to communicate will return to normal. While this may be true for some persons, communication problems will still exist for many individuals. A hearing aid cannot be expected to solve *all* of the communicative problems of the hearing impaired. If the major complaint of a person is difficulty hearing in noise, the problem may become worse when that noise is amplified through the hearing aid.

Fortunately for thousands of hearing impaired persons, the misconception that anyone with a sensorineural hearing loss cannot benefit from a hearing aid is dying a slow but certain death. The majority of hearing aids sold today are to individuals with sensorineural impairments. Their adjustment to a hearing aid may be difficult, but the rewards of improved communication may be the most gratifying.

Another misconception about hearing aids is that an individual can use any hearing aid as they all do the same thing; i.e. make sounds louder (Sanders, 1975). A hearing impaired individual should never purchase or wear a hearing aid given to them until it is first checked by an audiologist. This will assure that the hearing aid is appropriate for the type and severity of the hearing loss.

Optimistic advertisements have convinced many persons to purchase a hearing aid. This initial optimism, however, is often tempered by the realities of adjusting to the newly purchased aid. The hearing aid will benefit the user only in proportion to the willingness to accept the aid and to the patience and effort in learning to make the most of it (Silverman & Pascoe, 1978). Family and friends often make this acceptance more difficult by expecting too much too soon.

AURAL REHABILITATION

Ideally a new hearing aid user should be enrolled in an aural rehabilitation program. This type of program will generally emphasize not only the use of the hearing aid, but also the use of visual cues, such as mouth and facial movements during sound production, which can often compensate for short-comings of hearing aids (Hartford, 1979).

The nurse, because of close contact on a continuing basis with hearing impaired individuals, can become an integral part of this rehabilitation program. In aiding rehabilitative efforts of the hearing impaired, several suggestions will be helpful. These suggestions will benefit not only the new, but also the experienced hearing aid user.

1. Face the hearing impaired person directly and on the same level if possible.
2. Do not shout or exaggerate by increasing lip and facial movements. This will provide distorted and confusing information.
3. If a person has difficulty understanding something, find a different way of saying the same thing. Try to avoid repeating the same words over and over.
4. Keep your hands away from your face while speaking.
5. Never speak from another room or out of sight of the hearing impaired individual.
6. Be sure you get the person's attention before you begin to speak.
7. Reduce background noise (e.g. radio or TV) when talking.
8. Remember that a hearing impaired individual will not hear and under-stand as well when tired or ill.
9. Be patient! Successful communication is probably as frustrating for the hearing impaired listener as it is for the speaker.

In addition to following the above suggestions, the nurse has a unique opportunity to educate family members, medical staff, and other profession-als. Such education will certainly include the previously mentioned aids to communication for the hearing impaired and hearing aid care. Additionally, the nurse should stress to other significant individuals the need to provide the hearing impaired patient with opportunities to interact with those around them. The nurse should point out that it is not necessary for the hearing impaired individual to comprehend every word spoken to him or her. Get-ting the "gist" of a conversation and utilizing environmental cues will aid communication greatly.

The nurse, as a member of the health care team, can make a meaningful contribution to the hearing impaired individual. By serving in an educational and supportive role, the nurse will be able to draw the hearing impaired into contact with the hearing world. Too often, we allow these individuals to slip into a silent and isolated world. By working with, and caring for the hearing impaired individual, the nurse can be a powerful force in the support and carry-over of the audiologist's rehabilitative efforts.

REFERENCES

American National Standards Institute. *Specification for audiometers* (ANSI S3.6-1969: R1973). New York: ANSI, 1969.

American National Standards Institute. *Criteria for permissible ambient noise during audiometric testing* (ANSI S3.1-1977). New York: ANSI, 1977.

American Speech-Language-Hearing Association, Committee on Audiometric Evaluation. Guidelines for identification audiometry. *Asha*, 1975, *17*, 94–99.

Anderson, C.V. Hearing screening for children. In J. Katz (Ed.), *Handbook of clinical audiology* (2nd ed.). Baltimore, Williams & Wilkins, Co., 1978.

Bess, F.H. Impedance screening for children: A need for more research. *Annals of Otology, Rhinology, and Laryngology*, 1980, *89* (Suppl. 68), 228–232.

Gerber, S.E. *Audiometry in infancy.* New York: Grune & Stratton, 1977.

Giolas, T.G. *Basic audiometry including impedance measurements.* Lincoln: Cliff Notes, 1977.

Hartford, E.R. Guidelines for hearing problems: Substituting management for myth. *Geriatrics*, 1979, *34*, 69–72.

Jerger, J. Bekesy audiometry in analysis of auditory behavior. *Journal of Speech and Hearing Disorders*, 1960, *3*, 275–287.

Jerger, J., & Jerger, S. Diagnostic significance of PB word functions. *Archives of Otolaryngology*, 1971, *93*, 573–580.

Keith, R.W. Diagnostic audiometry. In R.W. Keith (Ed.), *Audiology for the physician*. Baltimore: Williams & Wilkins, 1980.

Maurer, J.F., & Rupp, R.R. *Hearing & aging: Tactics for intervention.* New York: Grune & Stratton, 1979.

Melnick, W., Eagles, E.L., & Levine, H.S. Evaluation of a recommended program of identification audiometry with school age children. *Journal of Speech and Hearing Disorders*, 1964, *29*, 3–13.

McCandless, G.A. Impedance measures. In W.F. Rintelman (Ed.), *Hearing assessment*. Baltimore: University Park Press, 1979.

Northern, J.L., & Downs, M.P. *Hearing in children* (2nd ed.). Baltimore: Williams & Wilkins, 1978.

Office of Demographic Studies. *Reported causes of hearing loss for hearing impaired students.* Washington, D.C.:Gallaudet College, 1973.

Rosenberg, P.E. The test battery approach. In J. Katz (Ed.), *Handbook of clinical audiology* (2nd ed.). Baltimore: Williams & Wilkins, 1978.

Sanders, D.A. Hearing aid orientation and counselling. In M.C. Pollack (Ed.), *Amplification for the hearing impaired* (1st ed.). New York: Grune & Stratton, 1975.

Silverman, S.R., & Pascoe, D.P. Counselling about hearing aids. In H. Davis & S.R. Silverman (Eds.), *Hearing and Deafness* (4th ed.). New York: Holt, Rinehart & Winston, 1978.

Skinner, M.W. The hearing of speech during language acquisition. *Otolaryngology Clinics of North America*, 1978, *11*, 631–650.

Wilson, N., & Walton, W. Identification audiometry accuracy: Evaluation of a recommended program for school-age children. *Language, Speech, and Hearing Services in Schools*, 1974, *5*, 132–142.

4

The Nurse and The Deaf Adult

Karen M. Jensen

INTRODUCTION

Medical care for the deaf patient is frequently a frustrating experience for both the patient and the medical staff. Many useful articles have been written about communicating with the deaf patient (Davenport, 1977; Golden & Ulrich, 1978; Heaster, 1975; Navarro & LaCourt, 1980; Sabatino, 1976). However, such publications seldom become meaningful until the health care professional is actually confronted with a patient who is deaf.

The Problem of Deafness

The patients being discussed in this chapter are those with a severe hearing loss or a profound hearing loss as described by Katz (1978) who cited Goodman (1965). Individuals with a *severe hearing loss* have an average hearing threshold level of 71 to 90 dB from 500 to 2000 Hz. They may be able to hear loud voices and environmental noises but are unable to hear consonant sounds. Such persons require special educational placement in programs for the hearing impaired.

Individuals with a *profound hearing loss* have an average hearing threshold level of greater than 90 dB from 500 to 2000 Hz, and may only hear very loud sounds. These persons do not rely on hearing as a primary channel for communication. In this chapter, we will oversimplify definitions, somewhat, and group these two hearing levels together. The term *deaf* includes those with a severe or profound hearing loss.

Because the congenitally deaf person does not have the opportunity to hear and absorb vocabulary and language as a child, the individual becomes very handicapped in the ability to use and understand the English language. Those who hear, learn the multiple meanings of words in our language by hearing them used repeatedly in context. The deaf child without this advantage often enters adulthood with only one meaning for any given word. It is, therefore, very important to recognize that the major handicap of deafness is not the inability to hear, nor is it the inability to communicate efficiently, but it is the inability to comprehend and effectively use language.

Case One—Barbara

Barbara has been deaf all of her life and had been diagnosed diabetic for 10 years. When her 2-week-old baby developed severe respiratory problems, Barbara immediately brought him to the hospital clinic in the town where she had recently moved. Because it is well-known that infants of diabetic mothers often experience problems in the neonatal period, the nurse in charge realized that it would be important to have a thorough prenatal history.

Because Barbara, the mother, was deaf, the hospital interpreter for the deaf was paged, and soon arrived at the clinic. Things went smoothly for the first few minutes while the basic history was taken. As the nurse began to present questions relating to the mother's diabetes, communication became more difficult.

The nurse asked, "Barbara, how often do you check your urine? Only once a day?" "Yes" Barbara replied. The nurse then asked "How does it usually run?" At this point the interpreter appeared to be somewhat confused. Barbara also looked confused, and the interpreter turned back to the nurse with a bewildered expression on her face. Not quite understanding the problem, the nurse reworded her question and asked, "How does it usually go?" The interpreter made an attempt to sign this sentence to Barbara, but obviously Barbara still did not understand.

At this point the interpreter turned to the nurse and said, "Could you explain what you mean?" The nurse then said "Well, is it +1 or +2 or what?" The interpreter signed this question to Barbara who then understood immediately and replied that it was +1.

The lack of communication in this situation resulted because the interpreter really was not familiar with the procedure of testing urine. When the nurse asked "How does it usually run?," the interpreter was at a loss because of not knowing how to interpret the word, *run*. The interpreter couldn't use the sign for *run* as in "running down the street," nor could she use the sign for *run* as in "the engine is running." The sign for a *run* in the stocking certainly would not have been appropriate. Fingerspelling the word *run* may not have solved the problem either, as it then would have been Barbara's responsibility to select which of the many meanings for the word *run* was appropriate in this situation. Very often, a deaf person such as Barbara will not have multiple meanings of a word in his or her vocabulary. The nurse should be prepared to encounter situations similar to the above.

The Deaf Population

Barbara is one of an estimated 13 million Americans who have a significant hearing impairment. Of this number, Shein and Delk (1974) have estimated that almost 2 million have such a hearing impairment that they cannot hear and understand speech. Of this number more than 200,000, like Barbara, lost their hearing before age 3, a critical period for mastering the English language.

The nurse may encounter deaf patients in a variety of settings but regardless of the situation the communication problems experienced will be relatively similar. The degree of difficulty experienced will often be directly related to two factors: The age when the patient became deaf and the degree of hearing loss.

The person who became deaf later in life may have very understandable speech. This individual may experience no problem with reading or writing, but may have great difficulty understanding spoken language. On the other hand, the congenitally deaf person like Barbara may have serious reading and writing weaknesses as well as unintelligible speech. This person will often be fluent in sign language, while the person deafened later in life may never learn sign language. The congenitally deaf person may have academic deficits as a result of the language handicap, while the individual whose deafness occurred later in life will usually have much more verbal knowledge and a broader vocabulary. The deafened individual will often have average communication with other family members, while the congenitally deaf person may have limited communication with family members who do not share the handicap of deafness. Emotionally, the deafened individual may experience serious adjustment problems and may also undergo personal career and family crises as a result of the sudden onset of deafness. The congenitally deaf individual may have made a normal psychological adjustment. The degree to which this occurs is, in large part, dependent upon the attitude of the deaf person's parents.

Hearing parents of a deaf child often experience great difficulty in accepting their child's deafness. They tend to question the potential of the child to become a normal productive adult; therefore, the child may grow up with a lowered sense of self-esteem. The deaf child of deaf parents, however, usually experiences full acceptance, without reservation. This child also has the advantage of greater exposure to deaf adults as role models, which helps to promote a more normal level of self-esteem and better psychological development (Witt & Ogden, 1981).

The ease of communicating with the hearing impaired person is usually related to the degree of hearing loss. The more hearing a person has, the better the individual's speech and language skills will be. The hard-of-hearing person will usually be more successful at understanding spoken conversations than will the deaf person.

As we concentrate primarily on the individual with a severe or profound hearing impairment in this chapter, it will become obvious that many of the principles involved also apply to the deafened patient and other hard-of-hearing patients.

Misconceptions

There are two common misconceptions about the deaf individual that nurses must dispel. The first is that most deaf people can understand speech through lipreading (often termed *speechreading*). While some exceptional deaf people are able to understand most of what is said to them by reading lips, the majority of deaf people in our society *do not* have this skill. They find lipreading difficult because of their language handicap. For example, it would be very difficult to successfully lipread the word *injection*, if one has only been exposed to the word, shot. Another problem affecting lipreading ability is the fact that about 40 to 60% of all English words look like other words when spoken on the lips. For example, the word *bed* looks identical on the lips to the words *pet, men, bet, met,* and *pen*. *Bed* also looks very similar to words such as *pat, pan, bad, mat, pit, pin, mitt, bit,* and *bin*. Even the best lipreaders understand only a small percentage of the actual words spoken. Good lipreaders have developed their ability through a thorough knowledge of the English language, and through the ability to correctly guess the identity of a spoken word from its context in the conversation.

The second common misconception is that deaf people can read and write English fluently. In a memorandum about communicating with hearing impaired patients, the American Hospital Association (Memorandum #12, 1978) reported that only about 12% of deaf American adults are proficient in English. Therefore, if the nurse relies on writing questions and messages to the deaf patient, the results may be discouraging. The average person who is born deaf or loses hearing before acquiring the use of language (prelingual deafness) reads English at a fifth or sixth grade level regardless of intelligence level. Written communication will have very limited effectiveness with such a patient.

Case Two—Carl

Carl had been hospitalized for 2 days, and appeared anxious and upset after a brief visit with his doctor. The nurse, who recognized Carl's fear, wrote him a note asking, "What is wrong?" Carl proceeded to show her a note written by his doctor. In it, the physician had attempted to explain that Carl would be taken for a liver scan that afternoon. Although his intentions were good, the doctor had not taken Carl's language limitation into consideration. The written explanation was far too difficult for Carl to understand, and it had produced anxiety rather than alleviating it.

The nurse was able to provide the reassurance Carl needed, by reading the doctor's note, and then rewriting the contents. "The man will give you dye. Dye is like red ink. You won't go to sleep. It won't hurt you. Don't move. They will take pictures. The man will tell you where to move."

The nurse's short sentences and simple vocabulary communicated the message, and Carl was very appreciative for the help. In addition, the nurse made arrangements for Carl's wife to accompany him when the procedure was scheduled. Having her available to assist in case of communication problems was very comforting to Carl.

We must realize that even though the deaf person may be handicapped in the ability to read and write as Carl is, this does not imply that the deaf person has limited intelligence. Deafness creates a handicap in the person's ability to learn English, but the person has normal ability to formulate and comprehend ideas. Therefore, the deaf patient must not be treated in a condescending manner as though mentally retarded. Deaf people have the same range of intelligence levels as people who can hear.

ETIOLOGY

Congenital deafness has several different causes. Knowledge of these etiologies may help the nurse in dealing with the patient and his or her family, which may include deaf parents and or siblings. In addition to direct patient care, the nurse may occasionally participate with the genetic counselor during genetic counseling sessions with deaf patients and their families. The nurse may also refer a patient for genetic counseling. There are three major types of genetic transmission of deafness: (1) autosomal dominant, (2) autosomal recessive, and (3) X-linked. Deafness is a major feature of several genetic syndromes.

Genetic counselors also deal with families when the cause of deafness is unknown or nongenetic. Prenatal exposure to certain viruses (rubella,

TABLE 4-1

Communication profile of the deaf patient*

Name _____ Address _____

Marital Status _____ Birthdate _____

Occupation _____

Medical information

Doctor _____

Previous hospitalization _____ Location _____

Previous surgery _____ Location _____

Corrected vision _____ OD _____ OS

Family or significant others

Name _____ Hearing _____ Deaf _____

Knows sign language: yes _____ no _____

How to contact _____

Name _____ Hearing _____ Deaf _____

Knows sign language: yes _____ no _____

How to contact _____

Communication style

Degree of loss: hard-of-hearing _____ profoundly deaf _____

Hearing aid use: _____ yes _____ no   Purpose of aid:

   Right hearing aid _____   Awareness of sounds _____

   Left hearing aid _____   Understanding of
                                        speech sounds _____

Speech _____ intelligible _____ unintelligible

Methods of communication

_____ signs _____ speech reading

_____ fingerspelling _____ gestures

_____ writing

Interpreter's name _____

How to contact _____

*NOTE: From "Communicating with Deaf Surgical Patients" by E.M. Wolf, *AORN Journal*, 1977, *26* (1), p. 43. Reprinted by permission.

cytomegalovirus) is a common cause of deafness and other handicaps. Frequently, children deaf due to an "unknown" cause are found to have a genetic form of deafness.

A very small percentage of deafness may be the result of other factors, including the administration of ototoxic drugs, blood incompatibility, and postnatal infections (meningitis, rubeola, and so on).

A more detailed explanation of etiologic factors is found in Appendix 4–A.

COMMUNICATION MODES

The aspect of most immediate concern to the nurse is communication with the deaf patient. Due to different educational approaches in the schools, deaf individuals do not all use the same means of communicating with the hearing world. To effectively deal with the deaf patient, the nurse must first know which type of communication the patient uses and prefers. Wolf (1977) has prepared a "Communication profile of the deaf patient" (Table 4–1), which if completed by the patient at the time of hospital admission and incorporated into the patient care plan, can greatly help to facilitate communication.

The communication profile clearly indicates that deaf patients do not all communicate in the same way. The wishes of the patient should be followed in selecting the most appropriate means of communication.

Oral Communication

As one becomes familiar with the field of deafness, two opposing philosophical schools of thought regarding the communication method that should be used in educating the deaf become apparent. One major group of educators feels that the deaf person will develop the best possible speech and lipreading skills if the individual is not introduced to fingerspelling or sign language. These educators emphasize speech, lipreading, and auditory training throughout the educational program. The deaf raised in such an oral philosophy may not know sign language or fingerspelling. For this reason, it is very important for the nurse to find out which type of communication the patient prefers. If the patient has been educated orally, a sign language interpreter might be useless. However, such a patient might request the services of an oral interpreter. An oral interpreter has been trained to speak clearly and to rephrase the conversation of a speaker to utilize the most visible vocabulary for the benefit of the patient.

The oral deaf patient may be able to lipread well enough to understand the speaker in most situations. However, the nurse caring for such a patient must realize when to *paraphrase* if the patient does not understand rather than repeat the same sentence in a louder voice. The nurse's face must also be visible to the patient at all times.

Case Three—Lori

At the age of 16 years, Lori (a very good lipreader) was hospitalized for a diagnostic workup for her cardiac problem. When she was scheduled for a heart catheterization, the nurse carefully explained the procedure to Lori and her mother. The nurse then watched as the mother paraphrased the explanation and told Lori what would happen. Lori appeared much less fearful after her mother's explanation, but still seemed tense and apprehensive the next day when she left her room for the procedure.

Due to the efforts of the nurse on Lori's floor, special arrangements had been made for the surgical nurse to remove her mask so that she could explain the doctor's directions to Lori. The nurse said, "Hold your breath," while pantomiming holding her breath, and said, "Okay, breathe," at the appropriate time. With this help, and a slight modification of hospital policy, the experience went smoothly and without anxiety for Lori, who was able to experience the procedure with the same degree of understanding and reassurance as any other patient.

Total Communication

Many deaf people have been educated in programs which advocate a total communication approach. Educators who advocate total communication feel it is to the deaf person's benefit to receive language input as early as possible. Therefore, the student is exposed to fingerspelling and sign language along with lipreading and auditory training. The patient who has been educated in a total communication approach will usually request the services of a sign language interpreter.

At one time or another we have all seen illustrations of the manual alphabet for the deaf. Many people do not realize that when the deaf communicate with each other, they do not spell out each word, letter by letter, using the manual alphabet. This would be much too cumbersome and time-consuming. Deaf persons use the manual alphabet in combination with signs that are movements representing whole words, phrases, or entire concepts. It is the combination of manual fingerspelling and sign language that composes the communication system used among most deaf adults. Table 4–2 shows the manual alphabet used in the United States.

There is currently more than one sign language system being used in the United States. For approximately the past 15 years, *English sign language* systems have been used in classrooms for deaf students. These systems, such as Signing Exact English (Gustason, Pfetzing, & Zawolkow, 1980) have attempted to provide the deaf child with an exact replica of the English

TABLE 4–2

The Manual Alphabet

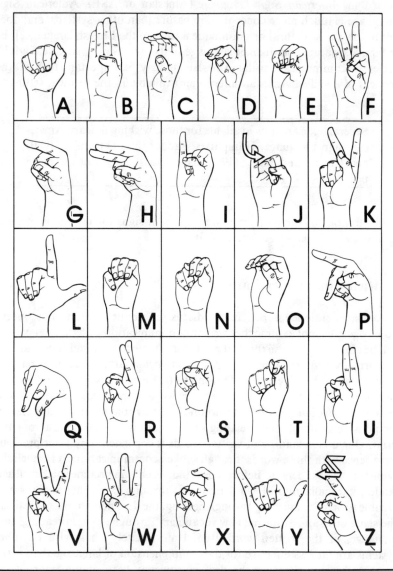

NOTE: From *A Basic Course in American Sign Language* by Humphries, Padden, and O'Rourke. Copyright 1980 by T.J. Publishers, Inc. Reprinted by permission.

language. Such systems utilize fingerspelling and sign language in combination with special signs representing verb tenses, plurals, and other grammatical prefixes and suffixes. While such English sign language systems are widely used in schools, communication between deaf adults is usually conducted in *American Sign Language* (Ameslan or ASL). American Sign Language is much more conceptual in nature than other systems, and does not follow the structural or grammatical rules of the English language. It is, in fact, a separate and distinct language of its own. Since many deaf adults prefer to communicate using Ameslan, it may be important to have the services of a skilled Ameslan interpreter available in the medical setting.

Several texts are now available for those wishing to learn American Sign Language. Humphries, Padden, and O'Rourke (1980) and Cokely and Baker (1980) have published two of the more popular books.

Illustrations of some of the more important signs for use in the medical setting are included in Appendix 4–B.

Written Communication

As was mentioned earlier in the discussion about common misconceptions, one must not assume that written communication with the deaf patient will be effective. Because the deaf patient is unable to hear and thus is unable to normally acquire language syntax and vocabulary, the level of reading ability may be relatively low. This might be more easily understood if you were asked to explain the meaning of the word *skragwobble*. If you had not seen a *skragwobble* before, and no one had ever told you what it was, you would have great difficulty relating to that word when you came across it in print. Our understanding of written words is dependent upon our previous experience with those words through spoken communication. It is much the same for the deaf person. Before a deaf individual can become successful as a reader, internalization of word meanings through experience is necessary. Unable to acquire meaning through hearing, the deaf person must substitute the sense of vision, acquiring new vocabulary through either lipreading, sign language, or the written word itself. Unfortunately, these visual symbol systems are far less effective for the comprehension of language than is the sense of hearing. Because the deaf person may have only a fragmentary understanding of the English language, it is natural for him or her to write in fragmentary and incomplete sentences. These written sentences may reflect the structure of Ameslan, which does not follow the syntax and structure of the English language, but has a unique conceptual structure of its own. Such sentences may seem awkward and difficult to understand as illustrated in the following situation.

Case Four—Cindy

Cindy, age 3½ years, was brought to the clinic by her deaf parents, Tom and Donna. They had both noticed that Cindy seemed to tire very easily. The parents were worried about the fact that Cindy seemed unable to play actively as long as her friends did. No sign language interpreter was available, so communication with the parents was attempted by writing notes. The nurse practitioner wrote several simple questions to Tom and Donna regarding birthdate, height and weight, and previous illnesses.

Donna communicated their concern about Cindy in a note that said "Cindy play tired breathe fast." Donna also pantomimed Cindy's behavior showing her breathlessness after vigorous activity. On examination the nurse practitioner detected an obvious heart murmur. The next question presented in writing to Tom and Donna was, "Does she ever squat?" This note bewildered them and they were unable to reply. They had never seen the written word "squat." All the parents could do was point to the written word and shake their heads, indicating they did not know what "squat" meant.

Understanding the problem, the nurse practitioner realized that the only way to get the concept across to the parents would be to act out the situation and demonstrate a child squatting after vigorous activity.

All medical professionals need to be aware of the limitation of using written communication with the deaf patient. Some patients and or their deaf parents will understand and be able to respond successfully. For these people, it would be condescending if we did not use writing to communicate. However, the majority of deaf patients will experience difficulty with written communication, both receptively and expressively. For these patients a skilled sign language interpreter is an absolute necessity.

The Sign Language Interpreter

Having available the appropriate interpreter would have prevented the occurrence of this somewhat humorous situation:

Case Five—Paul

Paul, a profoundly deaf dark-skinned Italian, was admitted to a hospital in central California for testing to rule out a possible ulcer. The admission procedure went smoothly, and Paul was shown to his room. Unfortunately, no one had bothered to notify the nurse on duty that Paul was deaf.

Soon after his arrival, the nurse entered the room and began by asking Paul several questions. When he tried to tell the nurse that he couldn't understand the queries, it was immediately realized that there was need to request an interpreter, which was done. In a few minutes, the interpreter arrived and began trying to talk with Paul. After a few minutes, the interpreter, realizing that Paul still did not understand, turned to the nurse and said, "I'm sorry, but I don't think this man speaks Spanish!"

Sub Section 84.52 (c), of HEW's Regulation under Sec. 504 of the Rehabilitation Act of 1973 (P.L. 93-112) states, "A recipient hospital that provides health services or benefits shall establish a procedure for effective communication with persons with impaired hearing for the purpose of providing emergency health care" (Memorandum #12, 1978—no page number). This requirement for hospitals to set up methods for communicating with deaf patients should be implemented not only in the emergency department, but elsewhere in the medical system where deaf patients may receive care; for example, in the eye clinic, hospital ward, orthopedic unit, physician's office, etc. (Memorandum #12, 1978).

Most hospitals have now attempted to comply with this public law, either by training one or more of their own personnel in the use of the sign language, or by compiling a list of locally available qualified interpreters. Due to the various types of sign language currently in use by the deaf population, and because of the complexities of communicating with a language-handicapped individual, we must guard against the temptation of using unqualified persons as interpreters. Most communities now offer sign language classes in churches, adult evening schools, and even in hospitals. However, successfully completing one or two sign language classes does not qualify one as a skilled interpreter. It usually takes several years of ongoing communication with the deaf population to produce a person skilled enough to interpret in the hospital setting.

The nurse who decides to study sign language can be of great assistance to the deaf patient. However, premature attempts to use such training in a medical situation should be considered with caution. The actions of the nurse who was on duty when Brad came to the emergency room illustrate this well.

Case Six—Brad

Brad, age 25, was admitted to the emergency room after suffering a severe blow to the head in a fight. The nurse on duty realized Brad was deaf when he did not respond to speech and pointed to his ear. The nurse had taken a sign language course, and was eager to use these limited skills. The nurse knew that Brad's hearing problem was probably not the result of his head injury, as he was totally conscious but unable to speak. He used his voice to make noises, but no one could understand him.

In sign language, the nurse asked, "Are you deaf?" Brad's face brightened enthusiastically, as he signed "yes," and began signing rapidly to the nurse. The nurse quickly discovered that she was unable to understand most of Brad's signs. Her beginning sign language course had taught English signs. The nurse assumed that Brad communicated only in American Sign Language (ASL). On a note pad, she wrote, "Do you know ASL" Brad wrote back, "All my life."

The nurse realized this patient would need an interpreter. The situation was a delicate one, in which Brad would have to respond to specific questions about his vision, tactile sensations, and so on. The nurse was able to contact the local organization of interpreters for the deaf and an ASL interpreter arrived at the emergency room within 45 minutes.

The nurse should be commended for recognizing personal sign language limitations and for knowing how to contact a qualified interpreter.

In 1980, a Seattle hospital underwent an investigation by the Federal Office for Civil Rights (OCR) when the mother of a deaf diabetic child filed a complaint claiming that effective communication was not available to her daughter who was admitted after experiencing a diabetic coma ("Needs of Deaf—", 1981). Investigators found that the emergency room staff was unable to communicate with the girl; written notes were unsatisfactory in such a situation; the sign language skills of trained hospital staff members were inadequate; and the hospital refused to hire a certified interpreter. The hospital was told to change its treatment of deaf patients or face the loss of federal funds.

The Registry of Interpreters for the Deaf is an agency that certifies qualified interpreters for various interpreting situations. The national office can direct you to your local chapter of Registry of Interpreters for the Deaf which can then suggest certified interpreters in your vicinity.

Registry of Interpreters for the Deaf
814 Thayer Avenue
Silver Springs, MD 20910

Telecommunication Devices for the Deaf

Deaf people are now able to communicate by telephone with other deaf people, family members, and friends through the use of telecommunication devices which look like small typewriters. Most of these devices are quite portable and many hospitals now have the equipment available for use by deaf patients. The machines are generally referred to as teletypewriters (TTY). The deaf person merely places the receiver of any telephone on the TTY machine and dials the number in the normal manner. If another deaf person who has a TTY is the call recipient, the telephone bell at this person's home will activate a light that alerts that person to the fact that the phone is ringing. When the receiver is picked up and placed on the TTY, the two individuals are then able to type their messages to each other across the telephone lines. The sender's device produces a series of tones that are then translated by the receiving unit into the typewritten letters that the receiving person can read from a display readout or a printout. The availability of the TTY in the room of a hospitalized patient can greatly improve morale and make the patient much more comfortable, and less isolated from family and friends.

Many hospitals have one or two portable TTYs available to place in patients' rooms, and, in addition, have another TTY permanently placed in a standard hospital location (such as at the switchboard or in the emergency room). This permanent TTY enables the staff to call a deaf person's home, and allows a deaf person to call the hospital for medical assistance or to set up appointments without having to request help from a hearing person.

Health care personnel should also be aware that many communities have services for the handicapped that provide a message service for deaf individuals in the community. If the medical facility does not own a telecommunication device, messages can be phoned to the local service agency which will then call the deaf person, using a TTY to convey the message. In reverse, the deaf patient using his or her TTY can call the service agency, explain the message, and the service agency will, in turn, call the medical facility to explain the request or concern of the deaf person.

For more information about telecommunication devices, contact:

Teletypewriters for the Deaf, Inc.
814 Thayer Ave.
Silver Springs, MD 20910

Gesture Communication

As very few health professionals know sign language, one of the best alternatives is communication through the use of simple, everyday gestures.

Most deaf patients will be able to readily understand gesture communication. This is because the deaf are very visually oriented, and for many of them gestures have become very important in communicating with the "hearing world." Deaf individuals from other countries are not familiar with the types of sign language used in the United States. However, communication between deaf Americans and foreign deaf individuals is seldom a problem. Deaf persons who use different sign language systems simply abandon both systems when attempting to communicate with each other, and revert to gesture communication, which is essentially universal.

The nurse will be greatly appreciated by the deaf patient when willing to dramatize and demonstrate information, rather than trying to communicate verbally.

Facial expression is extremely important to the deaf patient. If a face reveals worry or concern, the deaf patient may interpret this as meaning that his or her condition is worsening, or, perhaps, that the nurse is aware of and not disclosing some very negative information. The patient may arrive at this conclusion even though the concern expressed on the nurse's face is for another patient, or due to a situation completely removed from the work environment.

A very useful listing of some of the most helpful gestures is found in the chapter on nonoral communication.

The simplest, yet the most communicative gesture is a simple, caring touch.

Case Seven—Susan

Susan, age 62, was hospitalized for cancer treatment. A sign language interpreter was available for her at a scheduled time each day, but it was impossible to provide one fulltime. Most nurses avoided Susan. It was difficult and time-consuming to write notes to her, and often she did not understand the message. The nurses were uncomfortable with Susan's deafness and felt inadequate in communicating with her. They reacted by devoting their time to other patients whenever possible. Typical of many cancer patients who feel isolated and depressed, Susan's feelings were also compounded by her deafness and inability to communicate easily.

One nurse, Carol, decided to take a few minutes each day to provide what comfort she could to Susan. At first, she would sit at Susan's bed for just a few minutes each day and hold her hand or touch her arm. Susan's facial expression showed how much she appreciated Carol. After a few days, Carol decided she would try to communicate with

Susan through simple notes. Each morning she would touch Susan in some small, caring way, and write her a short, simple note, such as, "It snowed 4 inches last night. It is beautiful outside." It took very little of Carol's time, but it was the bright spot in Susan's day. Through the warmth of this simple touch and short note each day, Susan felt much less isolated.

Visual Media

The deaf patient will usually understand better if the nurse is able to use pictures, diagrams, or even handwritten illustrations in giving explanations. Whatever limited artistic ability the nurse may have to draw simple sketches will be appreciated. The patient will be able to understand drawings much better than might be expected. Three-dimensional models can be especially helpful in trying to explain anatomical structure as well as surgical or medical procedures.

Large index cards containing written common expressions will facilitate communication with the deaf patient. Such questions as: "Are you in pain?" "How are you feeling?" "Where does it hurt?" and "Would you like to go to the bathroom?" among others, can make communication with the deaf patient much faster and easier. A clipboard with lots of paper and a felt tip pen should be placed beside the patient's bedside at all times. If the patient wears glasses and or a hearing aid, be sure that they are within reach at all times. For some deaf patients with serious visual problems, it may be necessary to have a very large paper tablet and a broad-line felt tip pen available.

Additional Suggestions

Some of deaf patients' anxiety can often be reduced by allowing them to visit the various hospital departments where treatment will be provided. If it is known in advance that the patient will be sent to a certain department within the hospital for a specific procedure, it will comfort the patient to be taken there a day or so in advance. Then the environment will not be so frightening when the procedure must be performed.

Never restrict both arms of a deaf patient unless it is absolutely imperative for the patient's health. The hands of the deaf patient may be his or her only means of communication. By restricting movement, you risk severing the patient's only contact with his or her environment.

Lighting is extremely important to a deaf person. Don't leave the patient in a totally dark room—you have then rendered the patient "blind" as well as deaf. Also, avoid having your back to a bright light, as glare makes lipreading very difficult.

Flag the intercom button, the patient's chart, room, and bed so that all staff members will realize that the patient is deaf. Such notations should also mention the most effective way of communicating with the patient (writing, lipreading, or sign language).

RECOMMENDATIONS FOR THE NURSE

Some of the suggestions mentioned above are included in a complete set of guidelines for health care personnel which was developed at Gallaudet College located in Washington, DC, a federally funded college exclusively for hearing impaired students. These guidelines are reproduced in Appendix 4–C and provide a thorough description of procedures that should be followed during the hospitalization of a deaf patient. The guidelines are also very helpful in dealing with deaf patients in other health care situations.

COMMUNITY RESOURSES

Purpose and Function of Specific Community Resources

Depending on the circumstances, the nurse may wish to direct the deaf patient or the family of the deaf patient to one or more of the following resource agencies which are available in most communities.

1. *Registry of Interpreters for the Deaf*—This national agency also has state and local chapters which can provide a list of qualified interpreters in local areas.
2. *Vocational Rehabilitation*—State Departments of Vocational Rehabilitation maintain offices in most communities. These agencies are able to provide vocational counseling. They may also be of assistance in locating qualified local interpreters in communities with no local chapter of the Registry of Interpreters for the Deaf.
3. *Social Security Administration*—In certain circumstances, when the deaf person is eligible, on-going financial support can be obtained through the Social Security Administration.
4. *National Association of the Deaf*—This organization also has state and local chapters for the benefit of deaf individuals. It functions to meet the social needs of deaf persons. The Association is also very active in providing deaf persons with information of interest and importance to

them and is very active in seeking appropriate legislative action and legal services for hearing impaired persons.

5. *Alexander Graham Bell Association for the Deaf*—This organization promotes the oral approach to the education of hearing impaired children. It publishes a professional journal, *The Volta Review*, and sponsors local parent groups, and groups of oral deaf young people and adults. The national office is located at 3417 Volta Place, N.W., Washington, DC 20007.

6. *Community Service Agencies and Organizations*—Local organizations, such as the Kiwanis, Elks, Lions, and others, are actively involved in providing needed services for the handicapped. They often provide funding which is unavailable elsewhere to meet specific social or personal needs of the deaf.

7. *Speech and Hearing Agencies and Clinics*—Audiologists, who are qualified to recommend appropriate hearing aids, and speech-language pathologists, who are able to provide speech, hearing, and language therapy for the deaf individual, are often available within the hospital environment. They may also be found at local college and university clinics. Services in the area of speech-language pathology and audiology are also found in private clinics as well as through individuals in private practice.

8. *Genetic Counseling Clinics*—Qualified genetic counseling services may not be available in many small communities. Most genetic counseling centers are affiliated with medical facilities in large metropolitan areas. A directory of genetic counseling centers can be obtained by contacting any local office of the National Foundation/March of Dimes.

Locating Community Resources

Most local community services for the deaf can be located by contacting an experienced teacher of the deaf within the local school district. A more comprehensive way to locate services would be to consult the most recent April issue of the journal, *American Annals of the Deaf*. Each year, the April issue of this journal is a directory of all programs and services for the deaf in the United States. It includes educational and rehabilitation programs and services, as well as research and informational programs.

A complete listing of the contents of the April 1982 issue of *American Annals of the Deaf* is shown in Table 4–3. The annual April directory can be purchased by writing American Annals of the Deaf, 5034 Wisconsin Avenue N.W., Washington, DC, 20016.

TABLE 4–3

American Annals of the Deaf

Programs and Services
for the Deaf in the United States

April 1982	**CONTENTS**	Vol. 127, No. 2

Editors, Reference Issue: William N. Craig, PhD, and Helen B. Craig, PhD—
Western Pennsylvania School for the Deaf, Pittsburg, PA 15218. Reprinted
by permission.

CONCLUSION

The care and management of the deaf patient is both a challenging and rewarding experience. The patient and the health care professional may be equally apprehensive and anxious as treatment begins. However, with the use of the suggestions in this chapter the health care staff can minimize communication problems and reassure the anxious patients and families during treatment procedures. The results will usually be appreciative patients who are better able to cooperate during their own care and treatment.

ACKNOWLEDGMENT

This author gratefully acknowledges the assistance of Ronald Coles, LVN, Karen Epler, RN, Linda Miller, RN, Anne Ogden, RN, and Paul Ogden, PhD, who consulted in the preparation of this chapter.

REFERENCES

Cokely, D., & Baker, C. *American sign language*, Silver Springs, MD: T.J. Publishers, 1980.

Craig, W., & Craig, H. Programs and services for the deaf in the United States. *American Annals of the Deaf*, 1981, *126* (2), 87–316.

Davenport, S. Improving communication with the deaf patient. *Journal of Family Practice*, 1977, *4* (6), 1065–1068.

Dorland's illustrated medical dictionary (25th ed.), Philadelphia: W.B. Saunders, 1974.

Golden, P., & Ulrich, M. Deaf patients' access to care depends on staff communication. *Journal of the American Hospital Association*, 1978, *52*, 86–90.

Goodman, A. Reference zero levels for pure-tone audiometer. *Asha*, 1965, *7*, 262–263.

Guidelines for direct care staff. Washington, DC: National Center for Law and the Deaf, Gallaudet College, January 1980.

Guidelines for hospital policy for hearing impaired patients. Washington, DC: The National Center for Law and The Deaf, Gallaudet College, January 1980.

Gustason, G., Pfetzing, D., & Zawolkow, E. *Signing exact English.* Los Alamitos, CA: Modern Signs Press, 1980.

Hardy, J. Clinical and developmental aspects of congenital rubella. *Archives of Otolaryngology,* 1973, *98,* 230–236.

Heaster, P. Isolation isn't just a technique—Communicating with your deaf patient. *Journal of Practical Nursing,* 1975, *25,* 28–36.

Humphries, T., Padden, C., & O'Rourke, T. *A basic course in American sign language.* Silver Springs, MD: T.J. Publishers, 1980.

Jones, P. An educational comparison of rubella and non-rubella students at the Clarke School for the Deaf. *American Annals of the Deaf,* 1976, *121,* 547–553.

Katz, J. (Ed.). *Handbook of clinical audiology.* Baltimore: Williams & Wilkins, 1978.

Konigsmark, B., & Gorlin, R. *Genetic and metabolic deafness.* Philadelphia: W.B. Saunders, 1976.

Memorandum #12: Communicating with hearing impaired patients. Chicago: American Hospital Association, February 1978.

Navarro, M., & LaCourt, G. Helpful hints for use with deaf patients. *Journal of Emergency Nursing,* 1980, *6* (6), 26–28.

Needs of deaf not met by hospital. *Interpreter Views,* October 1981, p. 4.

Sabatino, L. Do's and don'ts of deaf-patient care. *R.N.,* 1976, *39* (6), 64–68.

Shein, J., & Delk, M., Jr. *The deaf population of the United States.* Silver Springs, MD: National Association of Deaf, 1974.

Witt, J., & Ogden, P. Politics and deaf people, part I. *The Deaf American,* June 1981, 5–8.

Wolf, E. Communicating with deaf surgical patients. *AORN Journal,* 1977, *26* (1), 39–47.

APPENDIX 4–A

ETIOLOGY OF DEAFNESS

Genetic Deafness

Konigsmark and Gorlin (1976) estimated that 35 to 50% of the cases of profound childhood deafness may be classified as genetic. As such a large percentage of the congenitally deaf population has a hearing loss attributable to a genetic etiology, we will briefly review the three major types of genetic transmission.

In *autosomal **dominant*** inheritance (the altered gene is located on an autosome rather than a sex chromosome), one parent usually passes on the gene. With each pregnancy the chances are 50% that the child will receive the gene for deafness from the affected parent. In addition, a mutation of a gene can occur at conception; in such a case neither parent has passed on the gene for deafness. Each individual deaf from dominant inheritance faces a 50-50 chance with each pregnancy that his or her offspring will also receive the gene for hearing impairment. Autosomal dominant disorders often vary in severity among affected persons. Therefore, the parent may have a mild or moderate hearing impairment while one of the offspring who inherited the same gene, might be born with a profound hearing loss. This phenomenon is termed *variable expressivity.*

Usually in families with *autosomal **recessive*** deafness, neither parent has a hearing loss nor do any other ancestors in either family. In this situation each parent carries the same recessive gene for the same type of deafness. However, because each parent also carries a normal gene, these parents are not deaf. When one of their children receives the same recessive gene for hearing loss from both parents, the child will be hearing impaired. It is important to keep in mind that there are many different recessive genes for different types of deafness. Autosomal recessive deafness will occur only when the recessive gene carried by each parent is identical in nature. Since, in most instances, deafness has not previously occurred in either of the parents' families, it is often difficult for these families to accept the fact that their child's deafness is genetic in origin. The explanation is that in prior generations, no family members ever married individuals who carried the same recessive gene for deafness. When both partners are recessive carriers, they have a 25% risk with each pregnancy of having a child who is deaf.

X-linked inheritance (the altered gene is located on one of the X chromosomes) only affects males. With this type of transmission the mother is a carrier who has normal hearing, but with each pregnancy in which the fetus is a male, the child will have a 50% chance of receiving the gene and being deaf. Of her female children, each will have a 50% chance of being a carrier as the mother. Men affected with X-linked deafness transmit the carrier state to all of their daughters but to none of their sons. In this condition there is never father-to-son transmission.

The type of genetic deafness in an individual is often not as clear-cut as it would seem by examining the three categories described above. This is because deaf individuals seek the company of others who are also deaf, forming a subculture that ultimately results in a great deal of intermarriage among deaf persons with varying types of genetic etiologies. We find many families with deafness throughout several generations, and in many of these families it is extremely difficult to determine what type or types of genetic transmission have been involved.

Of all forms of genetic deafness probably more than one-third of the cases are syndromal (Konigsmark & Gorlin, 1976). In individuals with syndromes, the deafness is accompanied by one or more additional physical characteristics. The additional identifying features may be of no serious medical significance, as in the case of Waardenburg syndrome. In addition to deafness this condition may include lateral displacement of the inner canthi of the eyes, patches of depigmented skin, a white forelock of hair, or a white patch of hair in another location on the head, and a difference in color between the two eyes (one eye being blue and the other brown, or occasionally both eyes being one color with one quadrant of one eye being another color). Other deafness syndromes can have serious medical implications, such as Usher syndrome, in which deafness is accompanied by retinitis pigmentosa (a progressive eye disease which can result in blindness). Jervell and Lange-Nielsen syndrome includes deafness and electrocardiographic abnormalities characterized by fainting spells and occasionally sudden death. Hundreds of deafness syndromes have been identified; therefore, it is important for the nurse to realize that most deaf patients should be seen for genetic counseling to determine whether or not important physical findings are present in addition to the deafness. Such accurate diagnosis can be important not only for the patient's own physical well being, but also for the well being of other family members who might want to have the information for purposes of family planning.

Teratogenic Deafness

A teratogen is an agent that causes the production of physical defects in the developing embryo (*Dorland's Illustrated Medical Dictionary*, 1974). The most common teratogens producing deafness in infants are viruses that attack the mother during pregnancy. Most of us are aware of the destructive effects of the rubella virus. Jones (1976) quoting Hardy (1973), reported that between 1963 and 1965 the rubella epidemic in the United States was responsible for the appearance of birth defects in 20,000 to 30,000 children, with up to half believed to have educationally significant hearing losses. In addition to deafness we now know that the rubella virus can also cause other serious physical involvements, such as mental and motor retardation, congenital heart defects, microcephaly, and visual defects. A large number of multihandicapped deaf children born during the epidemic of 1963 to 1965 are now approaching young adulthood. Professionals from all sectors of the health care system will find it challenging to meet the needs of this unique population in the years to come.

There are several other viruses that also have a teratogenic effect on the developing fetus. One is the cytomegalovirus. This virus is particularly insidious because the mother often remains totally asymptomatic during her infection. While the fetus is being attacked by the virus, the mother may experience neither a rash nor a fever to alert her to the presence of the virus. Cytomegalovirus can also result in deaf infants with additional physical and developmental handicaps.

Unknown

Many people are born deaf with unknown causes. It is suspected that a large percentage of these cases are actually genetic in origin. Autosomal recessive deafness usually cannot be identified until the birth of a second affected child in a family. If autosomal dominant deafness is the result of a new mutation, it is virtually impossible to identify it as a genetic form of deafness. Our medical and audiologic diagnostic procedures are not yet sophisticated enough to differentiate between the various etiologies of sensorineural deafness.

Appendix 4-B

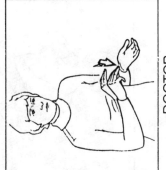

DOCTOR

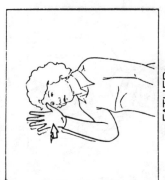

FATHER

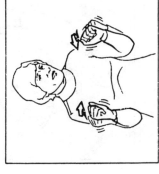

COLD, WINTER

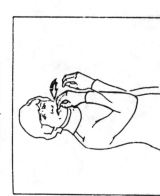

EAT, FOOD

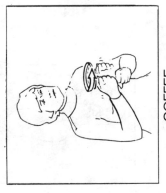

COFFEE

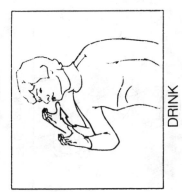

DRINK

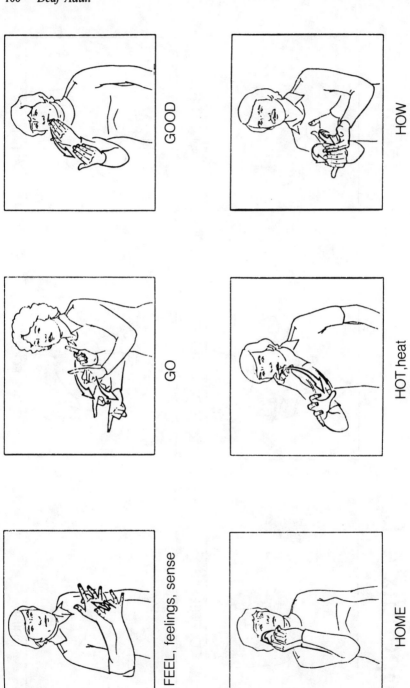

GOOD

HOW

GO

HOT, heat

FEEL, feelings, sense

HOME

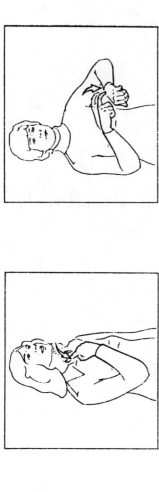

TIME

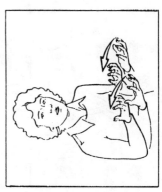

WANT, desire

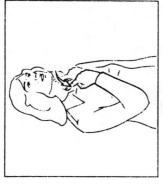

THIRSTY, thirst

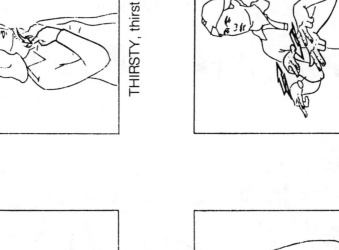

WALK

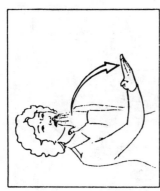

THANK-YOU

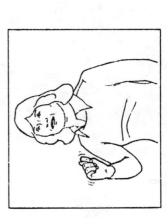

BATHROOM, TOILET

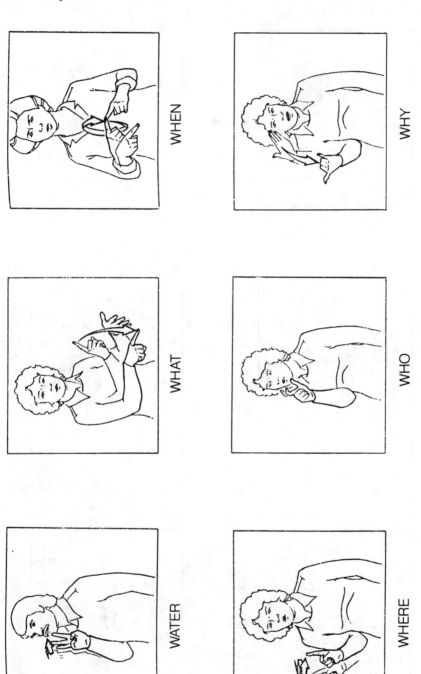

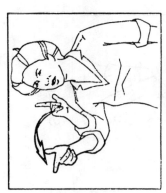

LATER

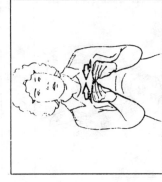

MORE, further

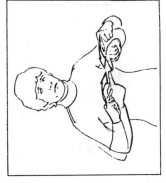

HURT, pain

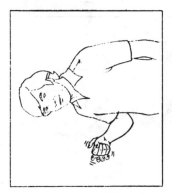

MILK

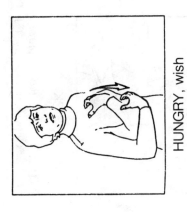

HUNGRY, wish

MEDICINE, chemical

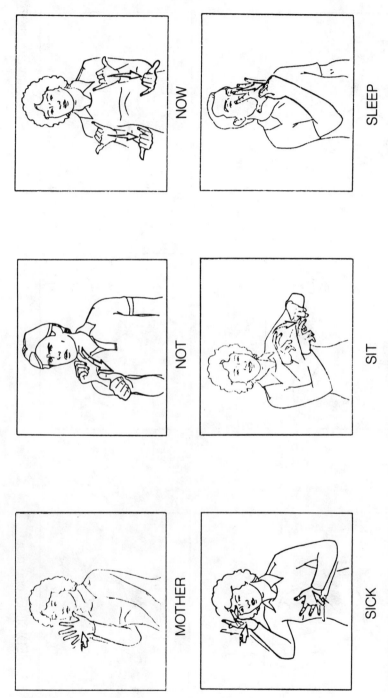

Appendix 4-C

GUIDELINES FOR HOSPITAL POLICY FOR HEARING IMPAIRED PATIENTS

    I. A central office should be designated to supervise services to deaf patients. This office should determine policy for provision of services to deaf patients, and staff knowledgeable about services should be available 24 hours a day. This office should be responsible for establishing and maintaining a system whereby qualified sign language and oral interpreters can be obtained on short notice 24 hours a day.

    II. The unit to which a deaf patient is admitted should immediately notify the designated office when a deaf patient is admitted.

    III. An interpreter, if available within the hospital, should be sent to the patient immediately to consult with the patient as to the patient's preferred method of communication, which may include:

        1. Use of qualified sign language and or oral interpreter
        2. Lipreading
        3. Handwritten notes
        4. Supplemental hearing devices, or any combination of the above.

        The interpreter should give the patient notice of his or her right to a qualified sign language and or oral interpreter to be provided by the hospital without charge to the patient, and to the deaf patient's right to a different interpreter if unable to communicate effectively with the interpreter provided.

        Should no interpreter be available within the hospital, the patient should be given notice of these rights in written form (at a reading level no greater than 5th grade), and be given the option of choosing one of the above methods of communication.

    IV. When an interpreter is the preferred method of communication, the interpreter assists in communications between the patient and hospital staff in all situations where effective communication is necessary to insure that the deaf patient is receiving equal services and equal opportunity to participate in and to benefit from hospital services. These situations include, but are not limited to:

        1. Obtaining the patient's medical history
        2. Obtaining informed consent or permission for treatment

3. Providing a diagnosis of the ailment or injury
4. Giving explanations of medical procedures to be used
5. Explaining treatment or surgery if the patient is conscious, or determining if the patient is conscious
6. Communicating during those times the patient is in intensive care or in the recovery room after surgery
7. Handling emergency situations that arise
8. Explaining the medications prescribed, how and when they are to be taken, and possible side effects
9. Assisting at the request of the doctor or other hospital staff
10. Discharging of the patient

   Friends or relatives of a deaf patient should *not* be used as interpreters *unless* the deaf patient specifically requests that they interpret. Deaf patients, their friends, and their families should be told that a professional interpreter will be engaged where needed for effective communication.

V. The deaf patient should be informed that another interpreter will be obtained if the patient is unable to communicate effectively with the assistance of a particular interpreter. The hospital shall obtain another interpreter if the patient indicates difficulty communicating with a particular interpreter.

VI. Any written notices of rights or services and written consent forms should be written at no greater than 5th grade reading level for deaf patients. An interpreter should be provided to assist if the deaf patient is unable to understand such written notices.

VII. A telecommunications device for the deaf (TTY) should be obtained and used for making appointments, for giving out information, and in emergency situations. Portable TTYs should be available on request for deaf inpatients.

VIII. Alternative methods of auditory intercom systems, paging systems, and alarm systems should be provided for hearing impaired patients.

IX. Ongoing efforts should be made by the hospital to sensitize staff to the special needs of deaf patients.

X. Contact with deaf people in the community, organizations for and of the deaf, and community agencies serving deaf people should be maintained for assistance in developing a list of qualified interpreters and in developing a program of hospital services that is responsive to the needs of deaf patients.

NOTE: Materials prepared by National Center for Law and the Deaf, 7th Street and Florida Avenue, N.E., Washington, DC, 20002. Reprinted by permission.

GUIDELINES FOR DIRECT CARE STAFF

There are many things individual hospital staff can do to aid in communication with a deaf patient, make the patient more comfortable in the hospital environment, and thereby give better services to the patient. Common sense combined with some basic information about deafness will aid hospital staff in providing good health care to deaf patients. It is important to remember that the deaf patient is the best resource and should be consulted for the preferred mode of communication and any problems that arise. The communication barrier between deaf and hearing people isolates deaf people and is overcome to the greatest extent possible by explaining to the deaf patient what is happening and answering any questions.

The importance of using a qualified interpreter to insure effective communication cannot be overemphasized. However, there may be routine situations (such as bringing dinner, checking in, taking temperatures, etc.) where an interpreter is not necessary. The following guidelines on working with deaf patients will help compensate for the absence of an interpreter when one is not present and will generally improve the quality of care provided.

I. Make added efforts in communication to insure the patient understands what is going on.
  1. Allow more time for every communication. Don't rush through what you want to say. Repeat yourself, using different phrases and be sure you have been understood.
  2. Don't exaggerate your lip movements. Speak at a normal rate of speed and separate your words.
  3. Don't restrict both arms of the deaf patient. Leave the writing hand free to write and sign.
  4. Make cards or posters of usual questions and responses that can be pointed to quickly.
  5. Keep paper and pen handy, but be aware of the wide range of English language fluency and writing skills found in deaf patients.

II. Be sensitive to the visual environment of deaf patients by adjusting lighting and using visual rather than auditory cues and reassurances.
  1. Use charts, pictures, or three-dimensional models when explaining information and procedures to deaf patients.
  2. Don't take a deaf patient's glasses away, or leave a deaf patient in total darkness.
  3. Avoid having your back to a bright light when communicating, as glare makes it difficult to read signs or lips.
  4. Face the patient when speaking and don't cover your face or mouth.

5. Keep your facial expressions pleasant and unworried. If you look like death is around the corner, the patient will be alarmed.

III. Alert all staff to the presence and needs of the deaf patient and be sensitive to those needs.
  1. Flag the intercom button so that workers will know the patient is deaf and requires a personal visit rather than a response over the intercom.
  2. Flag the patient's charts, room, and bed to alert staff to use the appropriate means of communication.

IV. Sensitivity to the special needs of people with hearing aids requires that hospital personnel:
  1. Always allow the patient to wear the hearing aid
  2. Do not shout at the patient
  3. Make sure that the patient has fully understood what has been said.

NOTE: Materials prepared by National Center for Law and the Deaf, 7th Street and Florida Avenue, N.E., Washington, DC, 20002. Reprinted by permission.

5

Management of Aphasic Stroke Patients

Nancy Helm-Estabrooks
Jennifer Chiavaras

INTRODUCTION

In this chapter we shall discuss the management of individuals with aphasia. Aphasia is an acquired language disorder resulting from brain damage. Because the ability to manipulate language is crucial to communication and communication is crucial to human interaction, aphasia compromises communication skills. The person with aphasia, therefore, may experience a devastating personal loss. The successful management of the language problems associated with aphasia depends greatly on what is known about the nature of the problem. This allows us to determine what can be done to compensate for the impaired language performance. The goal of aphasia treatment is to help patients maximize their potential for communication.

Acute Hospitalization

The brain lesion which produces aphasia often produces some physical symptoms requiring hospitalization. Earlier in this century a person with sudden onset of language disturbance may have been placed in a mental institution (Franz, 1906). Fortunately, aphasia is known now to be an unequivocal sign of brain disease rather than mental disease. As a result of our improved understanding, virtually all aphasic patients with access to modern medical personnel and facilities will be admitted to an acute care center for at least a period of evaluation. The length of the acute care hospitalization will depend on the complexity of the diagnostic workup and or on how sick the patient may be.

From the time of hospital admission to the time of discharge, the aphasic patient will be under the direct care of the nursing personnel. No other person will spend as much time with the patient. If the aphasic patient is to receive optimum care, the nursing staff must understand (1) the nature of the language deficits, (2) their psychological and emotional impact on the aphasic person, (3) the best methods for communication with these patients, and (4) the ways to maximize the potential for recovery. Studies of aphasia have shown that the period of greatest spontaneous recovery is the first few months post onset of stroke. It is during this time that therapeutic intervention is probably the most effective. The attending nurse is in a good position to assist in the recovery process, because the nurse spends more time than any other person with the patient during the spontaneous recovery period. In the absence of a staff speech-language pathologist, the nurse may be solely responsible for determining the most beneficial approaches to the patient with an aphasic disorder. When a speech-language pathologist is available, the nurse will be that person's greatest ally in carrying out the total language rehabilitation program.

Rehabilitation Centers

Aphasic patients with concomitant paralysis are often referred from the acute care hospital to a rehabilitation center. Although such centers typically employ speech-language pathologists, the nurse has the greatest contact with the patient. The responsible speech-language pathologist, therefore, will conduct inservice nurses' education sessions, enlist the nursing staff in a cooperative program of aphasia rehabilitation, and confer regularly with primary nurses regarding individual patients. The nurse also may be asked to monitor patient changes in on-ward communication during the course of formal therapy.

Nursing Homes and Chronic Care Facilities

Aphasic patients who are temporarily or permanently unable to return to their homes may be placed in a nursing home or chronic care facility. In many such facilities the nursing staff is totally responsible for the patient's ongoing rehabilitation program. Some chronic care aphasic patients may suffer from an active disease process such as arteriosclerosis, which has a poor prognosis. But even these patients with proper management may be able to maintain a functional level of language and cognitive performance for a longer period of time. For aphasic stroke patients with a stable medical status the prognosis generally is more favorable. Aphasic patients who live in a pleasant, stimulating environment may make continued slow progress indefinitely. Furthermore, recent research has shown that even patients with profound global aphasia may respond to a specific treatment program (Helm-Estabrooks, Fitzpatrick, & Baressi, in press). The nurse is often the person responsible for recommending and obtaining speech/language therapy services for chronic patients who begin to show a readiness and willingness for language therapy. Many patients who failed to improve with treatment in the early recovery stage may later become candidates for newly developed therapeutic approaches.

The Community

Some aphasic patients who return to their homes require ongoing nursing care for chronic disease such as diabetes or hypertension. Such patients may be seen in the home by the community nurse or in an outpatient clinic. For patients who are in an active outpatient aphasia therapy program the nurse may also become the liaison between the speech-language pathologist and the family. This is particularly true in communities which provide transportation for the handicapped individuals so that the speech-language pathologist has no direct contact with family members. A visiting nurse may assess the home environment, the family dynamics, and the functional communication skills of the patient. In fact, nurses often have more contact with the family than speech-language pathologists regardless of the setting. For example, in the inpatient setting a speech-language pathologist may miss family members who visit during the evenings. In such cases the prudent speech-language pathologist will call on the nurse for assistance in facilitating the role of the family in aphasia rehabilitation.

THE NATURE OF APHASIA

Cerebral Specialization

The language disorder called aphasia results from acquired brain damage. An understanding of aphasia is based on what is known of normal brain functions. In a circular fashion, much of our knowledge of normal brain/behavior relationships comes from the examination and study of persons with acquired brain lesions.

The human brain contains two cerebral hemispheres each controlling movement and sensation on the opposite side of the body. Damage to one cerebral hemisphere may cause weakness and or paralysis of the opposite side of the body. Weakness of the arm and leg on one side is referred to as hemiparesis; complete unilateral paralysis is called hemiplegia.

In addition to contralateral body control, the cerebral hemispheres have other specialized functions. The right hemisphere, for example, plays a greater role than the left in the processing of music and many visual-spatial concepts, while the left hemisphere is dominant for language in nearly all right-handed and the majority of left-handed individuals. This has been established through more than a century of clinical studies which have correlated left hemisphere damage with the disorder known as aphasia (Albert, Goodglass, Helm, Rubens, & Alexander, 1981). Each cerebral hemisphere is composed of four lobes: frontal, parietal, temporal, and occipital (see Figure 5-1) which also have specialized functions.

Aphasia Defined

Aphasia is an acquired, as opposed to developmental, impairment of the expression, manipulation, or understanding of language following brain damage. As a language disorder, aphasia differs from speech production disorders. Speech disorders are associated with damage of the neuromuscular apparatus which controls articulation and phonation. Patients with speech disorders may have intact language but have difficulty speaking the words. Aphasia also differs from the thought/cognitive/intellectual disorders which may accompany psychiatric or dementing diseases. We stress that aphasia is a *language* disorder and not a speech, emotional, or cognitive-intellectual disorder. Although patients with widespread brain disease may show all these symptoms as well as a language disorder.

Causes of Aphasia

Aphasia may be the result of cerebral-vascular accidents (stroke), traumatic head injury, tumors, infection, or degenerative disease. It is strokes, however, that are most likely to produce discrete unilateral left brain damage associated with aphasia uncomplicated by cognitive disorders such as loss of orientation in time and place. Cognitive disorders are more typical of individuals with widespread and or bilateral brain damage, although individuals with serious arteriovascular problems may experience multiple strokes affecting both left and right hemispheres.

FIGURE 5-1

Lateral view of the left hemisphere of the brain with middle cerebral artery and branches

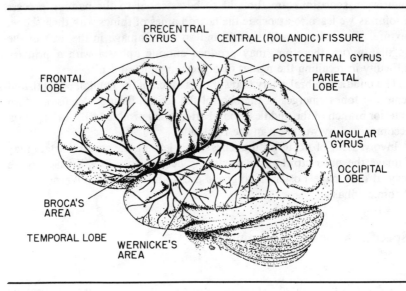

Neuroanatomical Basis for Aphasia

When aphasia occurs from left hemisphere stroke it may or may not be associated with hemiparesis or hemiplegia. Motor and sensory functions are controlled by the areas of the cerebral cortex immediately anterior and immediately posterior to the central rolandic fissure respectively (see Figure 5-1). The motor cortex is identified as the precentral gyrus; the sensory cortex is the postcentral gyrus. The movements and sensations of the opposite sides of the body are represented along these cortical gyri in an upside down fashion; thus, cortical regions for the face are located in the lower, or inferior, part of the gyri while the foot is represented superiorally (see Figure 5-1). Broca's area, responsible for encoding, that is to say producing or formulating speech, is located in the inferior portion of the 3rd frontal convolution immediately anterior to the cortical area representing the face. Damage to Broca's area will produce aphasia with primary deficits of verbal expression. Wernicke's area, responsible for decoding, that is interpreting speech, is located in the posterior portion of the first temporal gyrus. Damage to Wernicke's area will produce aphasia with primary deficits of auditory comprehension.

Another posterior area thought to be critical to language is located in the vicinity of the angular gyrus (see Figure 5-1). Geschwind (1965) refers to this as "the cross-modal association area" because fibers from auditory (temporal), tactile (parietal), and visual (occipital) reception areas of the brain all project to this region. Auditory-auditory, somesthetic-auditory, and visual-auditory associations are thought to be essential to the naming process insofar as we learn to associate the heard names of things with their shape, texture, size, color, smell, sound, and so on. Damage in the area of the angular gyrus, therefore, may produce anomic aphasia with a primary difficulty in recalling the names of objects, people, and places.

The middle cerebral artery that supplies much of the frontal, parietal, and temporal lobes emerges at the base of the central fissure. Occlusion of an anterior branch of the middle cerebral artery may produce a Broca's aphasia accompanied by weakness in the right side.

Involvement of posterior branches of the left middle cerebral artery may damage the postcentral gyrus producing hemisensory loss. Such a stroke may also damage posterior language areas and produce a Wernicke's or Anomic aphasia.

Specific Aphasia Syndromes

Aphasia is not an undifferentiated disorder. In fact, rather than speaking about aphasia, we should speak about the aphasias, because we can identify several specific aphasia syndromes which are manifest as distinct clusters of language behaviors. Clinical studies have correlated specific areas of brain damage with specific language behaviors and certain cortical and subcortical areas have come to be associated with certain aphasic syndromes. In this chapter we will describe only the major syndromes of aphasia. Albert, et al. (1981) may be referred to for descriptions of all known aphasia syndromes including those which occur with less frequency.

Anterior aphasia. Damage to areas of the brain anterior to the left rolandic (central) fissure will typically produce a nonfluent aphasia. Patients with nonfluent aphasia may retain relatively good understanding of incoming messages, but have sparse, effortful, poorly articulated verbal output. If the damage involves Broca's areas, the patient may manifest a distinct syndrome called Broca's aphasia.

Broca's aphasia. The following transcript was obtained from a Broca's patient who was describing a picture called "The Cookie Theft" (Figure 5-2) from the *Boston Diagnostic Aphasia Examination* (Goodglass & Kaplan, 1972).

FIGURE 5–2

"Cookie Theft" stimulus card from the *Boston Diagnostic Aphasia Examination*

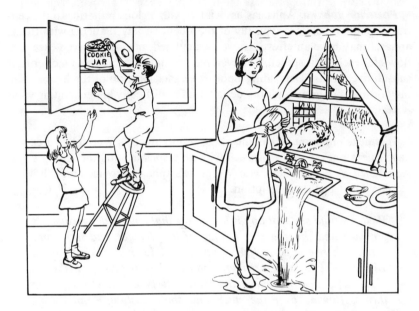

NOTE: From *The Assessment of Aphasia and Related Disorders*, Good-glass and Kaplan, Copyright (1972) Lea & Febiger. Reprinted by permission.

Mother's - ah - washin' dishes - but fauza [faucet] *- and ova* [over] *- flowin. Boy - stool - and fall. Cookies - and sister - and mother - day - - dreaming.*

Note that this description, although sparse, conveys a fair amount of information through the use of substantive (noun and verb) words. Unfortunately, these words are slowly and effortfully articulated so that the listener may grow impatient. The patient with Broca's aphasia does understand much of what is said to him or her, which facilitates communication.

Along with the language output deficit, a Broca's patient may have a right hemiparesis with more arm involvement than leg. Such a patient may have a functionless arm and hand but be able to walk with the help of a short leg brace and or cane.

Posterior aphasia. Aphasias associated with lesions posterior to the central rolandic fissure are typically of the fluent variety. Patients with fluent aphasia may have an effortless, well-articulated, normal, or even excessive flow of speech. This speech, however, may contain errors or may lack crucial substantive words. Depending upon the exact location of the lesion there may or may not be an auditory deficit, that is, difficulty understanding what is said.

Wernicke's aphasia. A patient whose lesion involves Wernicke's area will have fluent but error-filled speech with an associated auditory comprehension deficit. A male patient with Wernicke's aphasia provided the following Cookie Theft picture description.

> *Well, I would say that boy is falling off that fence—dangerous. He got hurt and the girl, too, falling off that hanger, and seen some cookies there and the coffee's going to fall down also. That's about all I can see in that picture there and here the girl is caught in the wet place here, doesn't realize that wet. The water is wetting from the—is flowing over the catch and she's washing - not paying attention to danger there.*

This rather lengthy description is misleading and confusing. The patient uses some wrong words like "fence" and "hanger" for stool. He inaccurately reports that the boy "got hurt" when the picture actually shows the stool merely in the process of tipping over. He uses excessive and imprecise language to tell us that the water is overflowing from the sink onto the floor and fails to state that the mother is washing the dishes while the children "steal" cookies. Indeed, the Broca's patient provided a better description with far fewer words.

In addition to the problems created by the confusing verbal output of a Wernicke's patient, communication is further inhibited by the patient's auditory comprehension deficits. Because Wernicke's aphasia is not associated with physical weakness as a visible sign of acquired brain damage, it was not unusual in the past for such patients to be considered psychotic. We now know that this is not the case, even though the patient may experience severe frustration.

If the posterior lesion spares Wernicke's area, the patient may have good auditory comprehension with speech that is empty of definite words, such as nouns. This syndrome is called Anomic aphasia.

Anomic aphasia. The following Cookie Theft transcript was obtained from a patient diagnosed as having Anomic aphasia.

> *Well, it's the - I know what it is, too, and I just can't—ah—well, they're getting ah—this thing here is the think—come—the—ah—I hate to say this, ah, but, I, I—ah—there's something over there— another house, no, that's not a house, I thought it was, but, but this is in—ah—it's—I know what it is.*

In many ways this description is the opposite of the one provided by the Broca patient, because it lacks the key substantive words which convey information. Instead, the patient is producing low information utterances, such as "I know what it is" and "I hate to say this" along with empty lead-in phrases such as "Well, it's the —." Indeed the anomic patient has told us even less about the picture than the Wernicke's patient who gave us some sense of what it depicted.

Like the patient with Wernicke's aphasia, the anomic patient typically has no hemiparesis. Because auditory comprehension is good and speech does not contain unusual or incorrect words, it is less likely that a patient with anomic aphasia would be incorrectly diagnosed as psychotic.

Aphasia involving anterior and posterior language areas. Massive involvement of the brain in the territory of the left middle cerebral artery may produce frontal parietal and temporal damage and thus injure all cortical language areas. The result will be a global aphasia accompanied by serious weakness of the right side of the body.

Global aphasia. Global aphasia involves all language modalities, so that the patient can neither produce nor understand spoken or written language. The ability to comprehend and produce symbolic hand gestures likewise may be impaired. Such patients may be reduced to the use of one real word, e.g., "boy, boy, boy," or meaningless stereotypical utterances, e.g, "bika, bika," which serve no communicative functions. Although the typical global patient will have great difficulty understanding spoken or written messages, some global patients have preserved ability to comprehend spoken commands that relate to axial (bilateral) movements, e.g. "Shut your eyes," "Stand up."

Psychological Reaction to Aphasia

The presence of language disturbances such as those described above can have a significant psychological impact on the aphasic individual. Benson (1973) reports that patients with nonfluent or anterior aphasias who retain the ability to comprehend language but have difficulty initiating speech are often visibly distressed and frustrated. Nonfluent patients, such as Broca patients, are more likely to be depressed than are patients with fluent posterior aphasias with auditory comprehension disturbance, such as Wernicke's aphasia. These latter patients may be unaware of their speech problems and therefore show inappropriate unconcern. Some patients with severe auditory comprehension disorders may think that other persons are actually talking about them, and this delusion may result in paranoia and perhaps impulsive or aggressive behavior. Unfortunately, this same auditory comprehension deficit makes counseling or psychotherapy difficult. Probably the most beneficial approach to the psychological reactions of any aphasic patient is to avoid isolation. Providing a group setting where patients meet others with similar problems may be helpful.

SPECIFIC ROLES OF THE NURSE

In the introductory section we stated that the role of the nurse vis-a-vis the aphasic patient is dependent somewhat upon the place and time of care. In an acute care hospital setting the nurse is likely to be among the first persons to see the aphasic patient. Immediate assessment of communication skills is crucial to patient management, particularly since the newly aphasic patient may have severely compromised language. The information gained from an assessment tool that identifies preserved channels of communication can be used to plan management strategies for both hospital staff and family members, which should reduce the emotional and psychological impact of aphasia.

By the time the patient has reached a rehabilitation center, his or her medical records will contain an aphasia diagnosis. Even so, the rehabilitation team will want to reassess the patient's communication skills because (a) different skills are needed for different settings and (b) patients may continue to change long after the initial insult.

An example of the first rationale for reassessment is illustrated by the Functional Communication Profile (Sarno, 1963) developed at the New York Institute for Rehabilitation Medicine. Among the skills this profile assesses is whether the patient can read his or her daily therapies schedule card and whether the patient can indicate the appropriate floor to the elevator operator. Although we sometimes use this profile in our institution, the patient's ability to perform these two communication skills can only be inferred. Our more independent patients must select and push elevator buttons themselves, there being no operators, while dependent patients are escorted to various therapies. All patient schedules are kept by ward personnel, so patients do not have to read a weekly schedule card, but instead are instructed as to where they next must go or are simply taken to appointments by the escort service. A complete assessment of our patients, therefore, includes a test of whether the seemingly independent patient actually understands either verbal or written instructions regarding his or her next appointment and whether the patient can select and push the correct elevator button to reach various departments within the hospital.

There is a large body of literature reinforcing the second rationale for reassessment, i.e. patients may continue to change over time. Although the greatest amount of natural spontaneous recovery of language may occur within the first few weeks or months post onset (Albert et al., 1981), most patients will continue to make small gains in communication over an extended period of time if the medical picture remains stable or improves. This is especially true for patients who have received language therapy or who have been in a stimulating environment. Sometimes these changes are not the result of improvements in primary language skills such as speaking, but rather are the result of learning to use compensatory mechanisms, such as gesturing and pantomime, facial expressions, and tone of voice. A patient who learns to add appropriate gestures and vocal expression to his or her limited verbal output, which may be a stereotyped expression such as "oh-oh," will become a better communicator than one who uses only limited verbalization. Because the nurse may be interested in evaluating the patient's ability to communicate within a particular setting at any point in time after onset of aphasia, a short assessment tool is required. The information obtained from this tool may then be used to plan management techniques for all persons who interact with the patient, including family and friends.

Assessment of Communication Skills

Anyone who attempts to assess an aphasic patient's communication skills must disavow themselves of the notion that communication is synonymous with spoken or written language. Although speech and writing are primary modes of communication, messages also may be transmitted through gestures, changes in vocal expression, and drawings.

Communication with gestures. Speaking and writing with accompanying understanding of spoken and written language are the primary means of communication for most people, but there are other ways to communicate— for example, the sign language of the deaf. Indeed, gestures are used constantly by all of us to communicate. These gestures have a wide range of sophistication. There are subtle unconscious expressions and movements called "body language," as well as hand movements we use to punctuate speech. There are deliberate, symbolic gestures such as the thumb to forefinger circle for "okay." Elaborate pantomimes are used by professional mimes, such as, Marcel Marceau, and gestures without spoken language may be used very effectively by construction workers or sports referees whose verbal signals may not be heard. Police control traffic with whistles and gestured signals which are decoded by drivers, and disgruntled drivers may signal each other with equally well recognized but less polite gestures.

Even severely impaired aphasic patients may appreciate gestures, and many aphasic patients retain all or partial ability to use gestures to communicate. Persons working with aphasic patients must remember this former fact at all times, realizing that gestures can be used to convey both negative and positive information. A person who makes circles around the ear with a forefinger to indicate "crazy" will probably be understood by even a globally aphasic patient who does not understand spoken or written language. (See Chapter 8 for a list of simple gestures.)

In an interesting study by Fordyce and Jones (1966) it was found that patients responded better to physical therapy tasks when given gestured instructions than when instructed verbally. We have found that some patients respond better to a combination of verbal and gestured instructions. These differences in findings may be accounted for by differences in the tasks to be carried out as well as possible differences in patient population. As stated, aphasia is not an undifferentiated disorder. Patients with various specific syndromes will differ from patients with another syndrome in communication skills which include production and appreciation of gestures. The point is one should explore every means of communicating a message to the patient, including the use of gestures.

Likewise, it is important to assess the patient's own ability to produce gestures. We have developed a nonvocal behavior rating scale which provides the frequency with which patients produce various gestures. This scale is rated by a variety of persons involved with the aphasic patient, e.g. nurses, speech-language pathologists, physical therapists, and so on. The speech pathology department used this scale in a pre- and posttherapy manner to note changes in patients' gestural skills with treatment, while nurses use the information to help determine communication strategies.

Communicating through prosody. The sounds and words that are combined for speech are called phonemes. Just as correctly combined phonemes are used to convey verbal information, so is prosody, or the "tone," of speech used to communicate messages. In English three prosodic features (rhythm, stress, and intonation) may be used to modify verbal messages. Sarcasm relies on prosodic changes. Taken at face value, a statement such as, "You're certainly artistic," said to a person who has just drawn a dog which looks like an anteater is either completely anomalous or says something negative about the speaker's art appreciation. But, with the addition of the appropriate suprasegment, that is, tone of the voice, the statement becomes sarcastic. There is growing evidence that patients with right hemisphere disease may have difficulty interpreting the suprasegmental aspects of speech, particularly those which convey emotion and humor, while those with left hemisphere disease and aphasia do not (Gardner, Brownell, Wapner, & Michelow, in press). Depending on their effect, suprasegmentals, or tones of voice, can be used beneficially to enhance communication with aphasic patients. Unfortunately, many reports on "how to talk with aphasic patients" advise speakers to slow down their speech. This is interpreted by some, and understandably so, to mean that one should prolong vowels or speak in a syllable-by-syllable fashion. This approach sacrifices many of the suprasegmentals which convey important information. A better approach is to use shorter utterances and longer interphrase pause time. Instead of saying "Mii-s-ter Jooones, pleeaase-stand-up-and grasp the wheel-chair-and-rotate-on-your-good foot," we recommend, "ok, stand up"—"good" "now, grab the chair," and so on, said distinctly and with enthusiasm.

An equally unfortunate bit of advice is that one should never speak loudly to aphasic patients. Although we do not advocate indiscriminate shouting, we remind the reader that aphasic patients are often elderly and may well have a hearing loss. An audiological examination includes tests of speech discrimination and loudness thresholds needed for understanding speech. If such an exam is not possible, the nurse can ask the patient to respond to spoken commands at various loudness levels. In addition, it is our experience that aphasic patients, like all of us, hear better if they can watch the speaker's facial expressions and lip postures. Whenever possible the nurse should speak to the aphasic patient face-to-face rather than behind his or her back or to one side. (See Chapter 3 for information on hearing impairment.)

Communication through drawing. Anyone who has seen Andrew Wyeth's *Christine's World* will agree that even a feeling may be communicated by a picture. Less artistic but highly communicative drawings are used commonly in our society. The button controlling the windshield wipers of your automobile may have a few straight lines and a raindrop depicted on it. A picture of a leaping deer on a road sign warns us that we are passing a deer crossing. Such pictures are iconic, that is, they look like the objects they stand for. Pictured symbols may also be arbitrary, for example, a circle with a diagonal bar has come to be associated with the concept "no," so that a drawing of a cigarette (iconic) surrounded by a circle and crossed by a diagonal line (arbitrary) communicates the concept "no smoking." Even severely aphasic patients may retain the ability to appreciate at least iconic or realistic pictures and drawings. In fact, a therapeutic approach for global aphasia developed by our speech pathology program begins with matching pictures to objects, because this skill is typically intact (Helm-Estabrooks, et al., in press).

FIGURE 5–3

Drawing of "Home" by patient with global aphasia

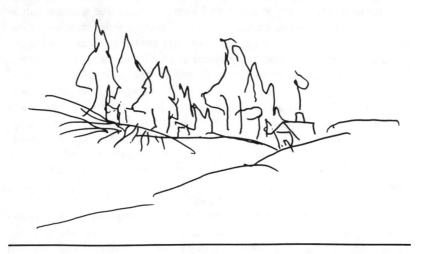

Likewise, some aphasic patients are capable of communicating by drawing, even in the face of severe agraphia (inability to write words). One such patient seen by us recently had a global aphasia with no ability to communicate through speaking or writing. When we asked where he lived and gave him a pencil and paper, he drew a picture for us (Figure 5–3). Although crude, it does convey the message that he lives in the north country. We correctly guessed Maine from his drawing. Another patient let us know he was constipated by drawing a toilet and a bottle of milk of magnesia.

Tools for evaluating aphasic patients' communication skills. Before the evaluation of an aphasic patient's communication skills, the nurse should be aware that the time is not appropriate if the patient has just been moved or is fatigued, confused, and or distressed. The formal evaluation is best done, therefore, in a quiet area after the patient has had an opportunity to settle in. Actually, the nurse begins to assess the patient's communication skills when meeting the patient. When the patient first arrives, we approach him or her with an outstretched hand and make a statement such as "My name is _____ and your name is?" We note if the patient attempts to shake hands or to say his or her name. This short introduction is followed by efforts to establish a trusting relationship with smiles and gentle touching which may be appreciated by even the confused patient. Basic security items such as bed, bathroom, and daily routine are presented along with introductions to fellow patients. We feel that the most important feature of a stroke unit is that patients have constant opportunity to interact with patients who may be worse or better off than themselves. This allows for mutual assistance, shared sorrows and victories, and the realizations that things could be worse and that they might get better.

Throughout the orientation period the nurse is informally evaluating the patient's communication skills. Once the patient has been oriented to the unit, the nurse can begin the formal evaluation of these skills. This evaluation will take about 15 minutes if the Boston Communication Assessment Tool (BCAT) is used. A BCAT evaluation is found in Appendix 5-A.

Planning Rehabilitation Approaches

The information obtained from the nurse's assessment tool and observations of nonverbal behavior can and should be used as a guide for determining communication approaches to the patient. If, for example, the patient can communicate better through writing or drawing than through speech, the nursing staff should provide pen and paper.

The information obtained from the nurse's assessment can also be shared with other staff members including the speech-language pathologist. It is not unusual for aphasic patients to respond differently to different environments. For example, the nurse may report that a patient diagnosed as globally aphasic from the speech-language pathologist's formal evaluation may understand most of the verbal and gestured commands given to him or her on the ward. The speech-language pathologist may use this information to help plan the treatment approach. Likewise, the nursing staff is often in the best position for noting change and progress in the patient's communication skills. This information should be relayed to the speech-language pathologist.

In order to assure a regular exchange of information we hold weekly chart rounds in which our patients are discussed briefly in terms of medical status, response to language rehabilitation, physical and occupational therapy, and their social and family situation. All staff members involved in the aphasic patient's treatment attend.

At St. Luke's Hospital in New Bedford, Massachusetts, where the nation's first acute care stroke program has been active since 1964, the weekly team meetings are attended also by homecare nurses from the surrounding communities. The goal of St. Luke's program is to return as many patients as possible to their homes. Before discharge, the visiting nurses assess the home environment so changes can be made, if necessary, to accommodate the aphasic stroke patient.

With or without team meetings it is the nurse who often serves as the liaison between all those involved in rehabilitation of the aphasic patient.

The nurse is most likely to regularly see the physician, speech-language pathologist, physical and occupational therapist, and family members and friends. In our hospital, visitors frequently visit in the evenings when only the night nurse is on duty. Our speech pathology program often relies on nurses to obtain information from the family. The nursing staff cooperates by asking families to fill out patient forms for the speech pathology program. One such form requests information on the patient's premorbid level of communication: talking, reading, writing, and television habits. This information helps determine rehabilitation goals. For example, we are not as likely to continue language therapy with a mildly aphasic patient who was quietly retired as we are with a patient who was a practicing attorney before the onset of aphasia. Without a good history we chance asking patients to perform beyond their premorbid level. For example, some patients may be unresponsive to a group approach or a ward atmosphere because they were premorbidly unsocial and not because of a reaction to the aphasia. This information is also important to the nurse who is responsible for assigning beds. Although it is our belief that aphasic patients do best in nonprivate rooms, knowledge of premorbid personality characteristics as well as postmorbid status may help determine how and with whom the patient is roomed. If possible, our patients are assigned to rooms according to severity and type of aphasia, so that a Wernicke's patient may be roomed with a Broca's patient or a mildly aphasic patient with a global aphasic patient. These placements usually assure a spirit of cooperation and assistance, alleviating some of the depression which may accompany the aphasia.

The Nurse as Counselor to the Patient

Previously we spoke of the nurse as a liaison between rehabilitation team members. The nurse, likewise, may serve as a liaison between the aphasic patient and other persons with whom she or he has personal contact. For example, the nurse may be aware that a patient dislikes one or more of his or her therapies and is resistant to leaving the ward for those appointments. Some patients prefer to work on one problem at a time. In our experience some stroke patients have been concerned more with walking than with talking. If the nurse makes the speech-language pathologist aware of this, the language therapy program may be scaled down until such a patient has begun walking and is ready to concentrate on language therapy.

Although the nurse may become aware of the aphasic patient's concerns simply through observation, our staff creates situations in which the patient can express feelings. Typically these situations are seemingly social and informal such as sharing a cup of coffee with the patient and asking how things are going. The first thing we hope this conveys to the patient is that his or her language problems do not make the aphasic less of a person. Secondly, we believe these contacts help the patient learn that there are legitimate reasons for being upset and frustrated. During these sessions, the patient is encouraged to express feelings. When the patient has difficulty verbalizing, the nurse can facilitate the process by putting some of the probable feelings into words for the patient, e.g. "It must be hard to be in the hospital," "You must be worried about...," "How do you like your food? I notice you didn't eat your..." Even if an aphasic patient is known to have great difficulty understanding speech, the ability to appreciate a friendly gesture, a tone of concern, or sympathy may be fully intact. Sometimes these situations allow the patient to simply have "the good cry" that the aphasic does not allow him or herself with family or therapists.

The Nurse As Family Counselor

Because of the nurse's central position on the stroke rehabilitation team, he or she is often the most likely person to engage in family counseling with full realization that aphasia is a family problem. In addition to interrupting or diminishing the flow of communication between the aphasic patient and significant others, aphasia often represents a permanent and drastic change in life-styles. When aphasia is accompanied by hemiparesis, even unskilled workers may be unable to return to former employment. When the former employment required easy manipulation of language, even mildly aphasic patients may be unable to resume their positions. These possibilities alone will have significant repercussions for the family in terms of finance and life-style. The nurse can assist the family during this difficult period by sharing information regarding the best means of communication with the patient, by referring the family to other team members including the social worker, and by allowing the family members to express their own feelings about the devastating loss, for aphasia indeed represents a loss. Families will experience fear, denial, anger, depression, and finally acceptance. In a sense they have lost as much as the patient. In fact, the patient may be so thoroughly involved in the day-by-day basic tasks of getting better that the family feels more helpless and hopeless than the aphasic. Often aphasia and or hemiparesis forces role reversals, particularly if the patient was premorbidly the dominant person, as in a parent and child relationship. With onset of stroke in the dominant individual, the "child" may be forced to assume the dominant, or parental, role. Unfortunately, family members often feel that they have no right to have or to express negative feelings because they do not have aphasia. The nurse can help the family verbalize these feelings, much as was done with the patient, e.g. "You must feel frightened by this," and so on.

To assist family members during the difficult period of hospitalization and rehabilitation we offer a family group meeting one evening a week. This meeting was originally organized by the nursing, social service, speech pathology, and neuropsychology services. There is always a representative from at least two of these disciplines in attendance. Family members are encouraged to express their fears and concerns that may include complaints about services being offered. Of course, one of the greatest benefits of these meetings is that these significant others no longer feel isolated, and they come to understand that feelings such as anger and depression are natural. These meetings also provide a forum for providing and discussing information regarding aphasia and hemiparesis, specific rehabilitative approaches, prognoses, and discharge plans.

The Nurse As Therapist?

In this chapter we have discussed the role of the nurse in the management of aphasic patients when there is also a speech-language pathologist as part of the rehabilitation team. The speech-language pathologist is responsible for developing and implementing all aphasia therapy programs. Obviously, there are situations where a speech-language pathologist is not directly available. Is the nurse in these cases responsible in some way for aphasia therapy? Our first instinct is to say that the nurse should never be responsible for any sort of formal language rehabilitation program because (a) the nurse is typically very busy with nursing duties and (b) the nurse does not have the necessary training for language rehabilitation. Just as a speech-language pathologist is not qualified to be a substitute nurse, a nurse is unqualified to be a speech-language pathologist. That is not to say that a nurse cannot carry out some routine aphasia therapy tasks under the guidance of a speech-language pathologist. In the absence of a nurse, a speech-language pathologist might be expected to manage and then refer a patient having a seizure or needing a bandage but would never hook up an IV. Likewise, in the absence of a speech-language pathologist a nurse may be expected to provide the optimal communication environment for a patient with severe auditory comprehension deficits but would not be expected to administer the Boston Diagnostic Aphasic Examination and develop a specific treatment approach. If a nurse is willing and able to carry out an accepted, appropriate, and pre-established language technique, however, it would be irresponsible to deny the patient this possible means of rehabilitation.

COMMUNITY RESOURCES

The nurse often acts as the primary referral person for the aphasic patient. This may involve simply telling the staff speech-language pathologist about the presence of an aphasic patient. If no staff speech-language pathologist is available, the nurse may review outside rehabilitation possibilities with family members. Most large metropolitan areas now have centers which offer total rehabilitation programs for aphasic stroke patients. If the patient is aphasic but not hemiparetic, then he or she may return home in need of outpatient speech and language therapy. Many large hospitals and some universities offer such services.

The best way to find out about community resources for speech and language therapy is to contact the:

American Speech-Language-Hearing Association
10801 Rockville Pike
Rockville, MD 20852

This organization can provide the names of agencies and certified speech-language pathologists in any area. Likewise, most cities have active speech, language, and hearing associations and or certified personnel listed in the yellow pages of local telephone directories.

For patients who are able to attend meetings, the Stroke Club International now has affiliates in most major cities. The objectives of this group's meetings are to assist stroke patients with problems of rehabilitation, employment, family, and community. The monthly meetings are conducted by professionals and stroke patients, themselves. Two publications, *The Stroke Memo*, a monthly, and the *International Stroke Club Bulletin*, a newsletter, keep members informed.

For further information contact:
Stroke Club International
805 12th Street
Galveston, TX 77550

The nurse may want to recommend or provide pamphlets for aphasic patients and family members. The following pamphlets may be obtained from:

American Heart Association
7320 Greenville Avenue
Dallas, TX 75231

Aphasia and the Family #50–002A
*Do It Yourself Again: Self Help Devices for the
    Stroke Patient* #50–005.A

Strike Back at Stroke #50–024.A
Strokes: Why Do They Behave That Way? #50–035.A
Strokes: A Guide for the Family #50–025.A
Up and Around Again #50–026.A

We also recommend:

Aphasia: Help Through Research #80–391, published by
Office of Scientific and Health Reports
National Institute of Neurological and Communicative Disorders
   and Stroke
Bethesda, MD 02005

ACKNOWLEDGMENT

Michael Alexander, MD, and Cheryl DiPaolo, RN, provided helpful suggestions for this chapter.

REFERENCES

Albert, M., Goodglass, H., Helm, N., Rubens, A., & Alexander, M. *Clinical aspects of dysphasia*. Wein, NY: Springer-Verlag, 1981.

Benson, D.F. Psychiatric disorders of aphasia. *British Journal of Psychiatry*, 1973, *123*, 555–556.

Fordyce, W.E., & Jones, R.H. The efficacy of oral and pantomime instructions for hemiplegic patients. *Archives of Physical Medicine and Rehabilitation*, 1966, *46*, 676–680.

Franz, S.I. The reeducation of an aphasic. *Journal of Philosophy, Psychology, and Science Methods*, 1906, *2*(23), 589–597.

Gardner, H., Brownell, H., Wapner, W., & Michelow, E. Missing the point: The role of the right hemisphere in the processing of complex linguistic materials. In Perecman, E. (Ed.), *Cognitive processing in right hemisphere*. Baltimore: University Park-Press, in press.

Geschwind, N. Disconnexion syndromes in animals and man. *Brain*, 1965, *88*, 237–294.

Goodglass, H., & Kaplan, E. *Boston diagnostic aphasia examination*. Philadelphia: Lea & Febiger, 1972.

Helm-Estabrooks, N., Fitzpatrick, P., & Barresi, B. Visual action therapy for global aphasia. *Journal of Speech and Hearing Disorders*, in press.

Sarno, M.T. *Functional Communication Profile*. New York: Department of Physical Medicine and Rehabilitation, New York University Medical Center, 1963.

Appendix 5–A

BOSTON VAMC COMMUNICATION ASSESSMENT TOOL

Patient's Name *D. F.*   S.S.#
D.O.B. 4-14-07   Phone:
D.O. Admission 9-28-81
D.I. Exam 9-29-81   Examiner: *J. Chiavaras*

Summary of Findings: *Good speech comprehension, fair speech production. Follows commands well. (see summary sheet)*

Materials: 8½" x 11" clipboard, 5" x 8" file cards with YES in large block letters and smiling face on one, NO and frowning face on other, medium felt tip pen, calendar, 2" adhesive tape, clock with movable hands.

Administration time: approximately 15 minutes

I. Information Processing and Orientation

PART A

Instructions: The following questions require a yes/no response. It is *not* necessary for the patient to say "yes" or "no." If verbal "yes" "no" is not reliable, explore pointing to yes/no cards, head nodding and shaking, raising and lowering arm, grabbing left arm of wheelchair where "no" card has been taped and right where "yes" card has been taped. Choose the most reliable mode of response and use it for the following questions.

Scoring: After all choices, score correct if the patient answers "yes" to only the correct item, that is the patient should answer "yes" to his or her name, to the right month, etc., and "no" to all other choices. Note the mode of response, e.g. verbal, head nodding, pointing.

Question	*Response*

1. Is your name _____
(provide multiple choice, making some choices phonetically similar, e.g. Don, *Dan*, Charles, John)

    Correct ___✓___

    Incorrect _____

    Mode of Response _*repeated his name*_

2. Is this an airport? a store? a hospital? a hotel?

    Correct ___✓___

    Incorrect _____

    Mode of Response _*said "yes"*_

3. Is this Beth Israel Hospital? the V.A. Hospital? the Mass. General Hospital? (give 1 correct and 3 geographically close choices)

    Correct ___✓___

    Incorrect _____

    Mode of Response _*said "yes"*_

4. Is this Jamaica Plain? Brighton? West Roxbury? Brockton? (give 1 correct and 3 geographically close choices)

    Correct ___✓___

    Incorrect _____

    Mode of Response _*said "yes"*_

5. Is this summer? winter? spring? autumn?

    Correct ___✓___

    Incorrect _____

    Mode of Response _*said "yes"*_

6. Is this May? June? April? December?   Correct _____✓_____
   (give 1 correct, 2 close, and 1 distant
   choice)   Incorrect _____

       Mode of   *said "yes"*
       Response _____

Level of information processing and orientation:

good (5–6) _____✓_____ variable (3–4) _____ poor (0–2) _____

PART B

Instructions: Regardless of the patient's score on Part A, test reading comprehension with a multiple choice format such as the ones presented below. Ask the patient to point to or circle the correct answer.

| **Stimulus** | **Response** |

1. My name is _____. (pick one)   Correct _____✓_____
   DON   DAN   CHARLES   JOHN
       Incorrect _____

2. This building is a _____. (pick one)   Correct _____
   AIRPORT STORE HOSPITAL HOTEL
       Incorrect _____✓_____

3. The month is _____. (pick one)   Correct _____✓_____
   MAY   JUNE   APRIL   DECEMBER
       Incorrect _____

Reading comprehension relative to speech comprehension:

Better _____ Worse _____✓_____ Same _____

II. Information Production and Orientation

Instructions: The following questions require the patient to provide information. If the patient cannot give a verbal response, ask for a written response, or drawing, or pointing to the calendar, or setting a clock, or holding up fingers, or selecting from a multiple choice. Note the content of the response (e.g. "Boston," "I don't know," "bika-bika") and the mode of response, (e.g., verbal, written, drawing).

Question | **Response**

1. Where do you live?

Response ___Hyde Park___

Mode ___spoken___

Correct __√__ Incorrect ____

2. Whom do you live with?

Response ___my wife___

Mode ___spoken___

Correct __√__ Incorrect ____

3. What is today's date?

Response ___29th___

Mode ___spoken___

Correct __√__ Incorrect ____

4. What time is it?

Response ___2 p.m.___

Mode ___spoken___

Correct ____ Incorrect __√__

5. How old are you?   Response ___24___

                             Mode ___spoken___

                             Correct _____ Incorrect __√__

6. What year were you born? Response ___1917___

                             Mode ___spoken___

                             Correct _____ Incorrect __√__

Level of information production and orientation:

good (5–6) _____ variable (3–4) ___√___ poor (0–2) _____

III. Following Commands

PART A

Instructions: Face the patient and ask him or her to act upon the following verbally presented commands.

Command	*Response*

1. Close your eyes   Correct __√_____

                             Incorrect _____

2. Stand up (accompanied with gesture; the   Correct __√_____
   hemiplegic patient just has to show he or
   she understands by trying to stand up)   Incorrect _____

3. Make a fist   Correct ___✓___

                                 Incorrect _____

4. Point to my nose   Correct ___✓___

                                 Incorrect _____

5. Look at the ceiling   Correct ___✓___

                                 Incorrect _____

6. Open your mouth   Correct ___✓___

                                 Incorrect _____

Ability to follow commands:
good (5–6) ___✓___ variable (3–4) _____ poor (0–2) _____

PART B

Instructions: If the patient scores in the 0–4 range on Part A, present the commands in printing and ask the patient to perform the movement.

Does the patient perform better to written than to verbal command?

Yes _____ No _____ Not Administered ___✓___

PART C

Instructions: If the patient scores between 0–4 to both verbal and written commands (Parts A and B) ask the patient to *imitate* the movements.

Does the patient perform better to imitation than to written or verbal commands?

Yes _____ No _____ Not Administered ___✓___

COMMUNICATION SKILLS SUMMARY

I. Patient's best mode of processing: *verbal*

Processing level with this mode:

good ___✓___ variable _____ poor _____

II. Patient's best mode of production: *verbal*

Production level with this mode:

good ___✓___ variable _____ poor _____

III. Patient's ability to follow *spoken* commands:

good ___✓___ variable _____ poor _____

If spoken not good then:

Patient's ability to follow written command:

good _____ variable _____ poor _____

If written not good then:

Patient's ability to imitate commands:

good _____ variable _____ poor _____

Instructions to Nursing Personnel:

This patient understands speech and verbal instructions well. He can read simple material. He has a lot of preserved speech, but if he can't say things he does well pointing to multiple choices. He can't communicate through writing.

6

Planning a Therapeutic Environment for the Communicatively Impaired Post Closed Head Injury Patient

Chris Hagen

A RATIONALE FOR NURSING INVOLVEMENT

The initial focus of treatment for the closed-head injury (CHI) patient is directed toward the existent life threatening and other physical injury conditions. An open airway and appropriate cardio-pulmonary function must be attained and maintained. Approaches to the control and monitoring of cerebral edema are instituted. Simultaneously, neurological and orthopedic surgery is often needed. Caught up in this activity is a distraught, anguished, frightened, and sometimes angry family who must also be assisted during this time of crisis. The intensity of nursing care is considerable. The pace of activity is quickened and the acute care treating team's responsibility is immense. All of these aspects of acute care are extremely dependent upon the expertise and judgement of a nurse. The need for this same level of nursing involvement continues even when the life-threatening conditions are stabilized and, ultimately, removed. While level and intensity of involvement remains the same in the post-acute phase of recovery, the type of nursing care becomes substantially different.

The most frequent handicapping residuals of CHI are of a behavioral rather than physical nature. Such injuries frequently result in some degree of impairment in the individual's cognitive-emotional/social-communicative abilities (Cronholm, 1972; Dye, Milby, & Saxon, 1979; Hooper, 1969; Jacobson, 1963; Lewin, 1966; Mandleberg & Brooks, 1975; Russell, 1932; Schilder, 1934). These areas of human function provide us with the basis from which to effect and maintain our self-esteem, relationship with others, and to actively pursue our vocational and avocational goals in life. In sum, it is our cognitive-social/emotional-communicative abilities that provide us with our means of leading a "meaningful" life. The meaningfulness of life is a measure of its quality. While the patient's physical life has been saved, we have only just begun the process of saving their mental-emotional-social life. If the physical existence of life is to have any meaning whatsoever in the broader context of human needs and values, then the eventual improvements in the quality of the patient's life must be addressed as quickly and vigorously as was the saving of physical life. Rehabilitation measures must be instituted as soon as, if not while, the life-threatening conditions are being stabilized. Consequently, the need for nursing care neither ceases nor does it simply become supportive once physical life is secure. On the contrary, the nurse must become an active participant in the rehabilitative effort. It is the nurse who plays the primary role in the initial phases of rehabilitation. The purpose of this chapter is to present guidelines and techniques for the nurse to enhance the speech-language pathologist's communication rehabilitation program for a patient.

CHARACTERISTICS OF COMMUNICATION DISORDERS

The CHI patient presents with a breakdown in communication abilities quite different from disturbances caused by vascular or space-occupying lesions. While these patients cannot understand or express themselves, they are not "aphasic" in the same sense that a stroke patient is "aphasic" because of a cerebral vascular accident. (See Chapter 5 for further information on aphasia.)

The CHI patient's communicative impairment results from the combined effects of disorganized and confused language processing and, if present, specific aphasic disorders. Further, the severity and nature of the patient's communication disturbance fluctuates considerably and randomly within a given day or across several days or weeks. At certain times they can be completely unresponsive though not comatose. At other times one may observe an outpouring of nonsense speech, but the patient's only response to the speech of others may be to turn toward the source of sound. On other occasions, the patients may understand bits and pieces of what is heard, and express themselves in fragmented and disjointed sentences composed of a combination of nonsense words, words that are only vaguely appropriate, and meaningful words with only portions of what is said being relevant to the patient's environment or the specific focus of discussion. As recovery continues, patients may begin to comprehend the general meaning of what has been said and be able to express their thoughts in sentences. The vocabulary used and the structure of their sentences may be accurate at this time, but they may fail to convey meaningful thoughts because their expressions are either irrelevant to the topic, confabulatory, circumlocutious, tangential, and or lacking in a logical order of related thoughts. During this time, the course of recovery of other patients may exhibit all of the characteristics of language disorganization noted above as well as signs of specific deficits in the ability to understand spoken speech and to express their own thoughts.

RELATIONSHIP BETWEEN NEUROLOGIC CONSEQUENCES OF CHI AND THE COMMUNICATION DISORDER

The presence and coexistence of confused language and specific aphasic disorders is a direct reflection of the effects of CHI on cerebral functions. The force of a blow to the skull is distributed to all parts of the brain. Thus, all parts of the brain suffer to a greater or lesser degree (Brain & Walton, 1969). At the moment of impact, the brain accelerates, rotates, compresses, and expands within the skull. The dynamics of these motions produce pressure waves within the brain substance (Brain & Walton, 1969; Feild, 1970; Walker, Kabros, & Case, 1944). All of these effects function to damage cerebral tissue through the dynamics of compression, tension, and shearing forces (Brain & Walton, 1969; Greenfield & Russell, 1963; Tomlinson, 1964; Walker et al., 1944). Compression forces tissue together. Tension pulls it apart, and shearing, which produces contusions and lacerations, develops at the points where the brain impinges on bony or ligamentous ridges within the cranial vault. Cerebral edema, which produces increased intracranial pressure, occurs shortly after this mechanical displacement and disruption of the brain substance (Meyer & Denny-Brown, 1955). In view of the magnitude and multiplicity of these negative forces, Russell (1932) and Adams and Sidmann's (1968) description of the effects of CHI as a "molecular commotion" appears quite appropriate. The very molecular structure of the brain is disrupted, disorganized, bruised, and or lacerated. These gross neuropathological effects of CHI have been found to produce permanent microscopic alterations of both white and gray matter. Brain and Walton (1969) report wide-scattered punctate hemorrhages throughout the brain associated with CHI. Severe localized demyelination was found by Greenfield (1938–39) but others (Strich, 1956; Tomlinson, 1964) have reported wide-spread white matter degeneration. Nerve cell damage after CHI has been reported both by Courville (1952) and Horowitz and Rizzoli (1966). Other permanent neurological impairments result from the contusions and lacerations of cortical tissue (Brain & Walton, 1969; Courville, 1942).

For additional information about other types of head injuries, see Rowbotham (1964).

The variety of the potential neuropathological consequences of CHI suggests that the initial generalized impairment of language/cognitive processes is a manifestation of the massive yet, to a degree, reversible disruption and disorganization of neurophysiological activity. Conversely the irreversible neurologic damage would, subsequently, produce a potentially wide variety of cognitive/language impairments that would not be expected to remit spontaneously.

While the severity of the irreversible neurological impairments often decreases during the first 3 months of recovery, their negative impact on functional language abilities continue for a considerable length of time. It has been my experience over the past 18 years with more than 2,500 head trauma patients to note that three general groups ultimately emerge from the diffuse symptomatology of the initial post CHI phase: (1) those with disorganized language secondary to cognitive disorganization who may or may not have a coexisting specific language disorder; (2) those with the predominant feature of a specific language disorder and coexisting minimal cognitive impairment; and (3) those with attentional, retentional, and recent memory impairments but without language dysfunction. The remainder of this chapter will focus on the treatment of patients who are in the first category, those whose primary communication disorder is one of language disorganization.

CHARACTERISTICS OF COGNITIVE-LANGUAGE DISORGANIZATION

Typically our internal and external environment is fluctuating, fluid, and random. Under normal circumstances we bring stability, structure, and organization to this otherwise chaotic world by automatically yet willfully focusing only on those things that we deem necessary and relevant to our needs. This ability to willfully focus our awareness on only certain aspects of our environment is derived from the following seven *cognitive processes*:

1. Attentional abilities (alertness, awareness, attention, attention span, and selective attention)
2. Discrimination
3. Sequential ordering of sensory stimuli and internal thoughts
4. Memory abilities (retention span, immediate, recent, and remote memory)
5. Categorization of sensory stimuli and internal thoughts
6. Association/integration of sensory stimuli and internal thoughts
7. Analysis/synthesis of sensory stimuli and internal thoughts

It is these seven cognitive processes that become disrupted in the face of CHI. Patients are unable to purposefully exert the influence of these processes on their internal and external environment. As a result, such individuals become disoriented, disorganized, confused, stimulus-bound, reduced in initiation, and reduced in inhibition. Consequently, the patient's receptive, integrative, and expressive language can also become:

1. Disoriented—not appropriate to the situation, question, statement, or discussion.
2. Disorganized—fragmented and incomplete understanding of what has been said or what the patient expresses.
3. Confused—confabulatory, circumlocutious, tangential in relation to the content of the situation, question, statement, or discussion.
4. Stimulus-bound—relevant to a part but not the whole idea of a statement, question, or discussion.
5. Reduced in initiation—reliant on others to stimulate the occurrence and structure of language responses.
6. Reduced in inhibition—once language response is initiated, it is lacking in specificity and precision in relationship to the original question or statement.

Typically, these six consequences of cognitive disorganization are seen in the patient's receptive and expressive language in combinations of the following symptoms:

(a) Decreased auditory comprehension;
(b) Decreased visual and reading comprehension;
(c) Expressive language that does not make sense;

(d) Language expressions that are grammatically correct but not relevant to the question, statement or discussion;
(e) Lack of ability to inhibit verbal expressions;
(f) Inappropriate ordering of words in sentences and or inappropriate grammar;
(g) Inability to recall specific words.

Many of these symptoms are characteristic of the aphasic disorders that are found in patients with vascular or space-occupying lesions. A CHI patient may, in fact, have a specific language disorder caused by a focal lesion. However, while many of these receptive and expressive language problems are like aphasia, the majority are symptomatic of the language confusion that results from the underlying disorganization of the seven cognitive processes listed above. While a significant portion of a patient's communication impairment is caused by *cognitive disorganization*, a major part of their communication rehabilitation program must be directed toward *cognitive reorganization*. As cognitive processes become reorganized, there will be a major decrease in the patient's language disorganization.

PLANNING A THERAPEUTIC ENVIRONMENT

The reorganization of cognitive abilities follows a predictable and hierarchial sequence (Hooper, 1969; Jacobson, 1963; Lewin, 1966; Russell, 1932) during which the patient, as described by Jacobson (1963) "....passes through the stages of mental development from intrauterine life onward through infancy, childhood..." and adult functioning. For this recovery process to occur, lower level cognitive functions must first be stimulated, stabilized, and reacquired. The reacquisition of lower level functions provides the basis for the activation, stabilization, and reacquisition of the next level of cognitive skills. To a certain extent, the subsidence of the mass neurological effects of CHI provides the spontaneous movement toward higher levels of ability. However, spontaneous neurologic recovery alone is not sufficient for patients to attain their highest post CHI cognitive/communicative potential. The rate, quality, and ultimate degree of recovery is critically dependent on the degree to which the environment and those within it interact with the patients at the threshold of their most intact level of cognitive abilities. Thus, while the neurologic sequalae spontaneously remit to a certain degree, the degree and quality of behavioral reorganization will be proportional to the degree to which the rehabilitation program purposefully channels spontaneous recovery, maximizes residuals, and helps the patient compensate for lost abilities.

The maintenance of a balance between the type and manner of all the patient's environmental stimulus input (e.g. auditory, visual, tactile, and so on) and their most intact level of cognitive functioning is the single most critical factor in the successful reorganization of cognitive/communicative abilities. Patients are able to process internal and or external stimuli in the most organized manner and, consequently, function at their optimum level of behavioral organization when the demands of the environment match their existing cognitive abilities. Environmental stimulation below the patient's most functional level will not challenge recovery in a structured, controlled, and predictable manner. Stimulation that is above a patient's current optimum level of cognitive functioning will be overwhelming and, as a result, will suppress and impede recovery.

Role of the Nurse in Establishing a Therapeutic Environment

Nursing personnel play a key role in the maintenance of a critical balance between a patient's best level of cognitive/communicative functioning and environmental demands that require the patient's utilization of those abilities. While it is important for all members of the treatment team to create and maintain this balance, it is the nurse who holds the potential of having the greatest impact on that balance. When one considers the patient's 24-hour day, it is clear that the nurse is the single member of the rehabilitation team with whom the patient has the greatest amount of interaction. The patient's course of recovery can be either positive or negative depending upon the type, nature, and quality of direct interactions with the nurse, as well as the general environment of the nursing unit.

The nursing unit is more than a place to provide ongoing medical care. It is more than a staging area in which the patient is prepared to go to treatment in other areas of the hospital. Everything that happens to and around the patient on the nursing unit has considerable therapeutic value. The nursing unit is a cognitive/communicative reorganization treatment unit. As such, there is as much of a need to plan the approach to treatment within this environment as there is in any other treatment environment. At a minimum, the planning of a cognitive/communicative therapeutic environment should be based on: (1) the patient's most intact level of cognitive functioning; (2) the speech-language pathologist's evaluation; (3) a knowledge of how to communicate with the communicatively impaired; and (4) a thorough nursing assessment. Additional psychosocial information provided by psychologists and clinical social workers is also extremely helpful.

Determining Level of
Cognitive Functioning

Historically, head trauma patients have been classified according to such categories as coma, stupor, delirium, and confusion (Lewin, 1966; Hooper, 1969). In recent years the Glasgow Coma Scale (Teasdale & Jennett, 1974; Jennett & Teasdale, 1977; Jennett & Teasdale, 1981) has also been extensively used. While the major purpose of the Glasgow Scale is the early prediction of mortality and morbidity, it also provides some very useful general descriptive categories of patient responses that are characteristic of different levels of coma. This scale is particularly useful during the acute care phase of treatment.

The Levels of Cognitive Functioning (Hagen & Malkmus, 1979) described in Table 6-1 have been found to be quite helpful in identifying a patient's most intact level of cognitive functioning throughout the entire course of rehabilitation. Unlike the Glasgow Coma Scale, the purpose of the Levels of Cognitive Functioning is not that of predicting prognosis. Its purpose is to assist in the identification of a patient's best level of functioning and, thereby, identify the best way of approaching the patient during the course of treatment.

The eight levels of cognitive functioning and behavioral responses in Table 6-1 form a hierarchy which has been observed to be characteristic of the behaviors of the CHI patient. By observing the type and nature of the patient's responses to the nursing unit environment and the responses to those who interact with the patients within it, one will find that behavioral responses characteristic of a particular level occur most frequently. For convenience in planning, patients are placed on the scale in relationship to their most frequently and consistently observed behavioral characteristics.

Most patients present a range of cognitive function which is characterized by a preponderance of behavior characteristics of one level and a scatter of behavioral responses below and above that level. Determination of the patient's range of cognitive/communicative behavior provides three types of information important to planning and maintaining a therapeutic environment; (1) Knowledge of the patient's most functional cognitive level identifies the highest level of functioning we can expect from a patient at a given point in time. Knowing this, the stimuli we present and the way in which we present them will not be below or beyond the person's capabilities; (2) Awareness of behavioral responses below the patient's most consistent level of functioning are extremely important in helping us know when the environment should be altered to maintain the patient's highest level of cognitive/communicative organization for the longest time possible. Behavioral responses characteristic of a lower level of function signal regression and as such tell us when to alter the way in which we are interacting with the patient or what we are

TABLE 6-1

Levels of cognitive functioning

I. *No Response*	Patient (P) appears to be in a deep sleep and is completely unresponsive to any stimuli presented.
II. *Generalized Response*	(P) reacts inconsistently and non-purposefully to stimuli in a non-specific manner. Responses are limited in nature and are often the same regardless of stimulus presented. Responses may be physiological changes, gross body movements, and or vocalization.
III. *Localized Response*	(P) reacts specifically but inconsistently to stimuli. Responses are directly related to type of stimulus presented as in turning the head toward a sound, or focusing on an object presented. The patient may withdraw an extremity and or vocalize when presented with a painful stimulus or may follow simple commands such as close your eyes, squeeze my hand, or extend an extremity, in an inconsistent, delayed manner. Once external stimuli are removed, (P) may lie quietly. (P) may also show a vague awareness of self and body by responding to discomfort by pulling at nasogastric tube or catheter or resisting restraints. (P) may show a bias toward responding to some persons (especially family; friends) but not to others.
IV. *Confused Agitated*	(P) is in a heightened state of activity with severely decreased ability to process information. (P) is detached from the present and responds primarily to own internal confusion. Behavior is frequently bizarre and non-purposeful relative to the immediate environment. (P) may cry or scream out of proportion to stimuli even after stimulus removal, may show aggressive behavior, attempt to remove restraints or tubes, or crawl out of bed in a purposeful manner. (P) does not, however, discriminate among persons or objects and is unable to cooperate directly with treatment efforts. Verbalization is frequently incoherent and or inappropriate to the environment. Confabulation may be present; (P) may be euphoric or hostile.
	Gross attention to environment is very short and selective attention is often nonexistent. Being unaware of present events, patient lacks short-term

TABLE 6–1 (continued)

recall and may be reacting to past events. (P) is unable to perform self-care (feeding, dressing) without maximum assistance. If not disabled physically, (P) may perform motor activities such as sitting, reaching, and ambulating, but as part of the agitated state and not as a purposeful act or on request.

V. *Confused, Inappropriate Non-Agitated*   (P) appears alert and is able to respond to simple commands fairly consistently. However, with increased complexity of commands or lack of any external structure, responses are non-purposeful, random, or at best fragmented toward any desired goal. (P) may show agitated behavior, but not on an internal basis (as in Level IV), but rather as a result of external stimuli, and usually out of proportion to the stimulus. (P) pays attention to the environment, but is highly distractable and lacks ability to focus attention on a specific task without frequent redirection by others back to it. With structure, (P) may be able to converse on a social-automatic level for short periods of time. Verbalization is often inappropriate; confabulation may be triggered by present events. Memory is severely impaired, with confusion of past and present in (P's) reaction to ongoing activity. Lacks initiation of functional tasks and often shows inappropriate use of objects without external direction. (P) may be able to perform previously learned tasks when structured, but is unable to learn new information. (P) responds best to self, body, comfort, and often family members. The patient can usually perform self-care activities with assistance and may accomplish feeding with maximum supervision. Management on the nursing unit is often a problem if the patient is physically mobile as he or she may wander off either randomly or with vague intention of "going home."

VI. *Confused-Appropriate*   (P) shows goal-directed behavior, but is dependent on external input for direction. Response to discomfort is appropriate and (P) is able to tolerate unpleasant stimuli (as NG tube) when need is explained. (P) follows simple directions consistently, and carries over tasks which have been relearned (i.e. self-care). (P) needs less supervision with old learning; ranges from unable to maximally assisted for new learning

TABLE 6-1 (continued)

with little or no carryover. Responses may be incorrect due to memory problems, but they are appropriate to the situation; (P) shows decreased ability to process information with little or no anticipation or prediction of events. Past memories show more depth and detail than recent memory. The patient may show beginning immediate awareness of situation by realizing he or she doesn't know an answer. (P) no longer wanders and is inconsistently oriented to time and place. Selective attention to tasks may be impaired especially with difficult tasks and in unstructured settings, but is now functional for common daily activities (30 min. with structure). (P) may show a vague recognition of some staff, have increased awareness of self, family, and basic needs (as food), but in an appropriate manner as contrasted with Level V.

VII. *Automatic-Appropriate*

Patient appears appropriate and oriented within hospital and home settings, goes through daily routtine automatically, but frequently robot-like, with minimal-to-absent confusion, but has shallow recall of what he or she has been doing. (P) shows increased awareness of self, body, family, foods, people, and interactions with the environment. Superficial awareness of, but lack of insight into, the condition is noted. Decreased judgment and problem-solving and lack of realistic planning for future. (P) does show carryover for new learning, but at a decreased rate and requires at least minimal supervision for learning and for safety purposes. (P) is independent in self-care activities and should be supervised in home and community skills for safety. With structure (P's) are able to initiate tasks such as social or recreational activities in which they now have an interest. Judgment remains impaired; such that (P) is unable to drive a car.

VIII. *Purposeful and Appropriate*

Patient is alert and oriented, is able to recall and integrate past and recent events and is aware of and responsive to the environment. Carryover for new learning is now evident. (P) needs no supervision once activities are learned. Within physical capabilities, (P) is independent in home and community skills, including driving, but may continue to show a

TABLE 6-1 (continued)

decreased ability, relative to premorbid abilities, in abstract reasoning, tolerance for stress, and judgment in emergencies or unusual circumstances. Social, emotional, and intellectual capacities may continue to be at a decreased level but functional in society.

---

requesting of the patient; (3) In a similar fashion, recognizing the emergence and stabilization of behavioral responses characteristic of the next highest function level alert us it is safe to alter the environment to challenge the patient to move toward this next level of function. It is on the basis of this information, i.e. patient's most functional cognitive level, responses below and above that level, that one is able to construct the type of environment that will maintain cognitive organization. The ideal nursing unit environment is one that presents stimuli to match the patient's most stable level of functioning, simultaneously challenging the next highest level of functioning. By matching and slightly challenging the patient's best level of functioning, the environment and those within it function to decrease the behavioral swings below the patient's most intact level and increase the frequency and degree of swings above it. Soon the patient will begin to function all the time at the next highest level. Then one will discern a scatter of responses remaining from the previous level and the beginning of abilities at the next highest level.

Patients at or between Levels III and VII may fluctuate considerably in their range of functioning. Such fluctuations may occur from hour to hour or from day to day. In order to know a patient's most functional level at any given time, it is helpful to have all disciplines rate the patients at the time they treat them. Figure 6-1 presents a charting method that has been found to be useful. The observers enter their initials or the initials of the discipline in the box marked examiner, the time and the date of observation are entered in the boxes at the top right, and a check is placed in the box opposite the behaviors that were observed. This rating sheet should go with the patients throughout the day to all of their appointments. In this way those who are receiving the patient from the nursing unit will quickly know how to approach the patient and, conversely, the nurse will know how to adjust the approach and the environment when the patient returns to the unit throughout the day. This is quite critical in that the patients' level of functioning while on and off the unit may be very different from that exhibited when they return. Sometimes patients will be functioning at a lower level and sometimes at a higher level than when last seen by a nurse. If the nursing approach is based solely on a patient's level of functioning when last seen, there is the potential of handling the patient at the least

FIGURE 6–1
Level of Cognitive Functioning Record

Patient: _____ Date of Birth: _____

Date of Onset: _____

Diagnosis: _____

√	Examiner	Department	Time	Date

VIII. *Purposeful-Appropriate*

   a. Alert, oriented; intact recall for past and recent events.

   b. Demonstrates carryover for new learning; functions independently, within physical capabilities, once new tasks are learned.

   c. Able to formulate realistic goals for own future; may be candidate for vocational rehabilitation.

   d. Able to apply adequate judgment to daily living and community situations relative to premorbid ability level.

VII. *Automatic-Appropriate*

   a. Appropriate and oriented within hospital-home settings.

   b. Able to go through daily routine with minimal-to-absent confusion; depth of recall may be shallow, however.

   c. Demonstrates carryover for new learning although at a decreased rate; requires at least minimal supervision for learning and for purposes of safety.

FIGURE 6–1 (continued)

	Examiner	Department	Time	Date

d. Demonstrates superficial insight into disabilities, decreased judgment and abstract reasoning; lacks realistic planning for own future. Prevocational evaluation and counseling may be indicated.

VI. *Confused-Appropriate*

a. Inconsistently oriented to time and place; recent memory is impaired with decreased detail and depth of recall.

b. Follows simple directions consistently; responses are appropriate but may be incorrect if requiring recent memory.

c. Supervised for new learning with little or no carryover but shows carryover for previously learned skills.

d. Actively participates in therapy programs and demonstrates some purposeful behavior but remains dependent on external structure.

V. *Confused-Inappropriate-Non-Agitated*

a. Alert, demonstrates gross attention but difficulty maintaining selective attention.

b. Demonstrates severe impairment of memory functions.

c. Responses are fragmented and frequently inappropriate to the situation, reflecting confusion and lack of goal-direction.

FIGURE 6–1 (continued)

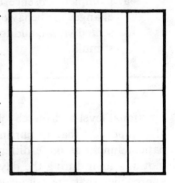

d. Demonstrates agitation in response to external stimuli.

e. Wanders from treatment areas.

f. Absent carryover for purposes of learning; assisted to maximally supervised in activities.

IV. *Confused-Agitated*

a. Alert and in heightened state of activity but demonstrates severely decreased ability to process environment. Responds primarily to own internal agitation.

b. Performs motor activities but behavior essentially non-purposeful relative to environment.

c. Demonstrates aggressive or bizarre behaviors.

III. *Localized Response*

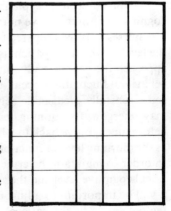

a. Demonstrates withdrawal or vocalization to painful stimuli.

b. Turns toward or away from auditory stimuli.

c. Blinks when strong light crosses visual field.

d. Follows moving object passed within visual field.

e. Responds to discomfort by pulling tubes or restraints.

f. Responds inconsistently to simple commands.

II. *Generalized Response*

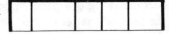

a. Demonstrates generalized reflex response to painful stimuli.

FIGURE 6–1 (continued)

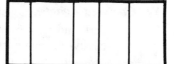

✓	Examiner	Department	Time	Date

b. Responds to repeated auditory stimuli with increased or decreased activity.

c. Responds to external stimuli with physiological changes.

I. *No Response*

a. Complete absence of observable change in behavior when presented visual, auditory, or painful stimuli.

---

functional level and thereby precipitating cognitive disorganization. It is also important that all nursing shifts participate in this process. Often a patient functions quite differently during the evening, night, and early morning than during the day. During those times one may need to use approaches that are completely different from those taken during the daytime.

As can be seen, the planning and implementation of a therapeutic cognitive/communicative nursing unit environment is a dynamic process. The nurses must be prepared to make frequent changes and adjustments in the level at which the patient is expected to function, the way in which they approach the patient, and in the overall environment of the unit. Although behavioral fluctuations occur, this type of serial rating will begin to identify some generally predictable behavior patterns. For example, some patients may emerge as functioning best early in the morning, regress considerably before lunch, move back to a higher level in the afternoon, but not as high as the morning level of functioning, and then regress slightly in the evening. In order to maintain the critical balance between the patient's most functional cognitive level and the stimulus demands of his or her environment, it will be important to adjust the environment and your interactions with the patient to fit the patient's most functional level at any given point in time. By rating and charting behaviors, the nursing staff will rapidly become aware of a patient's general pattern of functioning. Knowledge of the patient's pattern is very important for environmental planning. With daily behavioral information one will, within limits, be able to predict the patients' most intact level of function at a particular time of day and, often, in relation to certain nursing unit activities. With this amount of predictability, the nursing staff will be able to plan in advance the best way of approaching the patient throughout all shifts.

Utilization of the Speech-Language Pathologist's Information

The speech-language pathologist's diagnostic evaluation will typically encompass the patient's abilities in: comprehension of spoken speech, comprehension of written material, ability to mentally formulate thoughts into words, verbal expression of thoughts, written expression of thoughts, coordination and control of muscles involved in speaking, arithmetic, and the level and nature of cognitive functioning. The results of the evaluation not only provide the speech-language pathologist with information that is used to determine the type, nature, severity, and prognosis of the patient's communication disorder, but also give the nurse critical information. For example, the speech-language pathologist's report will indicate the patient's best channel (i.e. auditory or visual) through which to present instructions, questions, or statements. From the report, the nurse can also determine whether the patient should be expected to communicate verbally, and, if so, to what extent.

Some specific examples of how the nurse can use the information obtained from the speech-language pathologist are:

1. If a patient has extreme difficulty in understanding spoken speech but has little difficulty in understanding visual signs, as many instructions as possible should be given through *gestures, pictures,* and *demonstrations.* Use of spoken words only distracts and confuses this patient, making it difficult to use his or her visual mode of comprehension for greatest efficiency. For instance, when teaching wheelchair-to-bed transfer, the maneuver should first be demonstrated by the nurse. One should actually sit in the wheelchair and demonstrate all of the positions and the maneuvers involved in the transfer. It helps also if one breaks the transfer process down into a number of easily observable steps and repeats each step several times before proceeding to the next. Then the patient should attempt the different steps. If the patient becomes confused and forgets a step, that step is shown again. This procedure is used until the patient can perform consistently and accurately all of the steps involved in the transfer.

2. If the patient has a minimal-to-mild deficit in understanding spoken speech, the same procedure is used as above. However, this patient's learning can be implemented by using *1 or 2 concrete words when demonstrating each step*, rather than by talking in strings of sentences. For example, when teaching the patient to lock a wheelchair, say, "Lock chair." This is more helpful than "Now, George, I want you to lock your wheelchair first before you do anything else," which could thoroughly confuse the patient because you have given too many words to try to understand and you have given two ideas to think about. Visual signs paired with a simple phrase help this type of patient learn both visually and verbally.

3. If the patient understands spoken speech but has a severely decreased auditory retention span, it is important to give him or her only one instruction at a time. Sufficient time must be allowed for a response before the next instruction is given. Since decreased auditory retention span is quite frequent in head trauma patients, it is a good rule to *give instructions singularly rather than sequentially*, regardless of the degree to which the patient understands. Because of difficulty with retention, it should never be assumed that the patient will remember instructions from one moment to another, or from one day to the next. With this problem, it is helpful if the manner in which instructions are given does not vary from moment-to-moment or day-to-day. If there is a change in the manner or the content of the instructions, the patient becomes confused thinking the he or she is being asked to do something completely new and different.

4. If the patient has difficulty in understanding spoken speech but can read, the second procedure in this list is used. A printed word, instead of a spoken word or two, is employed when demonstrating the different steps. The words must be printed large enough to compensate for any peripheral visual problem the patient may have.

5. If the patient cannot understand spoken speech, visual demonstrations, pictures, or words, then the approach should *only be through physical demonstrations*. The nurse should actually move such a patient through the different steps of the task and then immediately stimulate him or her to repeat what was done. This is done by moving the patient through the first several steps and then encouraging the patient to complete the remaining steps of the task. Then the number of steps provided by the nurse should be gradually decreased until the patient can follow through on the complete task in response to a request.

While five different types of patients and possible ways of communicating with them have been given, it must be remembered that these are only illustrative and do not necessarily represent all of the combinations of communication problems that occur in head trauma patients.

IMPLEMENTING A THERAPEUTIC ENVIRONMENT

Strategies for Management of Cognitive Dysfunction

The importance of adjusting the nursing unit environment relative to fluctuations in the patient's level of cognitive/communicative abilities was stressed earlier. There are, however, general treatment strategies that are applicable to specific levels of functioning regardless of the needs of a particular patient. For this purpose, the eight levels can be condensed to four.

Levels I, II, and III: No, generalized and localized response. The goal of treatment for Levels I and II is to activate a behavioral response and thereby initiate the patient's movement toward the early phases of awareness of his or her environment.

Activation of behavioral responses will occur within the context of routine nursing care of the patient. Special efforts outside of this routine do not have to be taken. The stimulation of the patient toward Level III will, however, be enhanced by giving special consideration to the manner in which the nursing routine is carried out. The following ways of interacting with patients hold the potential for stimulating the patient's awareness of the environment.

1. Be calm and soothing in manner of speech and physical manipulation of the patient;
2. Do not talk to others when working with the patient;
3. Assume the patient can understand all that is said. While it will be unknown at this time the degree to which the patient can actually understand, it is wiser to not run the risk of patients hearing comments about themselves or other patients. When such conversations are heard and understood, it can be emotionally traumatizing and create emotions that have the potential of affecting the future course of recovery. Consequently, all comments or discussions of the patient's medical status, behavior, discussion of prognosis and family concerns as well as discussions about other patients should be conducted in another area;
4. Talk to the patient. It is quite difficult to carry on a conversation with an unresponsive patient, however, try to avoid the feeling that since the

patient cannot answer there is not much point in talking to him or her. Talking is a natural form of stimulation. Use appropriate greetings such as "good morning Mr. or Mrs. Smith." Describe what you are going to do with the patient before you do it, describe such occurrences as family visits, upcoming occupational therapy treatment, and so on, talk about the weather conditions or even things or events that are of personal interest to you. Try to learn about the patient's family and or friends so that you can talk about them by name and describe some of the things they are doing. However, it is important not to overwhelm the patient with talking. Talk slowly and calmly. Describe what you are about to do with the patient then, without talking, do it and then describe the next event. It will be important to leave moments of silence between verbal stimuli.

5. Manage environmental stimuli. While activation of the patient's behavioral responses at these lower levels is dependent upon the presence of external stimulation, too much stimulation can suppress movement toward awareness of environment. A TV or radio is a very useful source of stimulation. However, it is important to have one on at random times and for short durations. The patient will rapidly get used to and not respond to such stimuli when one is on continuously. It will also be necessary to have only one source of stimulation in the environment at a time. For example, if talking is occurring, then the radio or TV should be off.

6. Determine which type of stimuli seem to cause the patient to respond. Certain topics, statements, TV programs, music, and so on may elicit a response. Often family voices or voices of a particular staff member seem to stimulate a response. In the case of these latter two possibilities, tape recordings can be made of those to whom the patient reacts and played intermittently to the patient. When key stimuli are identified, present them to the patient on a routine basis. However, the patient will become fatigued and overwhelmed if such stimuli are allowed to continue for long periods of time. To a large extent, arousal and awareness depend upon the novelty of the stimulus. All such activities should be kept very brief. It is better to present several different types of stimuli than to present the same one too long.

7. Encourage the family to follow the same pattern of interaction as outlined above. Special caution should be taken to describe the problems of presenting simultaneous multiple stimuli and stimulating the patient for too long a period of time. If not helped to understand the problems, the family can unknowingly overwhelm the patient.

Level IV: Confused-agitated. The goals for this level are to increase the patient's awareness of and attention to the environment, minimize the frequency of agitated behavior and when agitated behavior occurs, decrease its duration.

The physical handling and moving of patients as well as your manner of interacting with them is most important at this stage. The patient is beginning to be aware of and alert to the environment and is trying to process information. The neurological status at this time, however, is such that there is often an exaggerated response to internal and external stimuli. Thus, a patient at this level is very susceptible to the triggering of defensive motor reflexes and emotional reactions such as acute fear, anxiety, and anger. Many of these behavioral responses occur spontaneously and are unavoidable but special efforts taken by the nurse can minimize the degree and duration of such responses. Some of these responses are avoidable. However, the degree to which one is able to keep from triggering the patient's defensive responses is the degree to which the patient will be in a neurological position to move towards the environment rather than away from it. Approaches to take with patients at this level include:

1. Be calm and soothing in manner when handling the patient;
2. Move slowly around the patient and move the patient slowly when it is necessary to change the person's position or range or bathe or transfer the patient;
3. Talk slowly and softly. Loudness will trigger a startle reflex and rapid speaking rate will be overwhelming;
4. Do not talk to others while working with the patient. Multiple stimuli such as physical manipulation and an ongoing conversation with others will be more than a patient can handle;
5. Always describe what you are going to do with the patient before you do it. Even if what you say is not totally understood by the patient, the time it takes to explain things will give him or her time to adjust to your presence in the room and to become aware that something is going to happen;
6. Before physically handling the patient for a desired task, take time to first simply touch the patient, gently rub one of the extremities, head, or back and or gradually move an extremity. Such activities will decrease defensive motor reflexes and emotional reflexes—allowing the patient time to adjust;
7. If the patient becomes upset, allow time for self-adjustment. Do not try to talk a patient out of his or her reaction. At this time, talking will be an additional external stimulus that will only act to intensify the reactions;
8. If the patient remains upset, either remove him or her from the situation or remove the stimuli;

9. Watch for early signs that the patient is becoming agitated (e.g. more than usual motor movement activity, increase in vocal loudness, resistance to activity) and modify the environment immediately. It is far better to cease all of your activity than to launch the patient into a prolonged state of agitation. It will take far less time to wait than it will to calm the patient down.

Levels V and VI: Confused, inappropriate non-agitated and confused appropriate. The goal of this phase of rehabilitation is to create the environmental conditions whereby the patient can produce purposeful and appropriate responses to external and internal stimuli with greater frequency and duration. There are two approaches to creating the appropriate conditions. One involves the use of the more automatic behavioral responses found in some of the activities of daily living. Such activities can be used as a means of eliciting purposeful behavior and provide environmental structure. Activities of daily living such as dressing, eating, toilet, and leisure time tasks provide numerous opportunities to gently challenge a patient to move toward purposeful and appropriate responses. For example, putting a pant leg or shirt sleeve partially over one extremity but not over the other encourages the patient to complete the task. Rather than allowing the patient to randomly attempt to organize the act of teeth brushing, the nurse can stay with the patient and lay out the various components of the task in the appropriate order and help him or her move stepwise though each component of the task sequence. Meals can be structured in the same manner. In essence, any and all routine tasks that a patient carries out on the unit can be turned into cognitive reorganization tasks. All that is needed is to recognize the tasks as such, then assist the patient by breaking the tasks into subcomponents, initiate the first step or two for the patients, and maintain the patient's structure in proceeding through the task. If the patient begins to become confused, the nurse can intervene and assist in initiating the next appropriate behavioral response in the sequence and then withdraw, allowing the patient to continue. On the surface, this nursing approach would appear to have the potential of consuming a tremendous amount of time per patient at a time when all on the unit are extremely busy with a multitude of responsibilities. However, confused patients left to their own devices will actually require more time from nursing. Such patients do not complete tasks, or complete them partially or inappropriately. They begin to wander around and off the unit and are prone to handle objects and materials in a manner that creates work for others. The patient who was told by the nurse to get dressed and start toilet activities and then left alone only to be discovered later flushing clothes down the toilet while mumbling something about a "washing machine" will be long remembered by both the nurse who had to search out new clothing and start all over again with the patient as well as by the maintenance person who had to take the toilet apart to retrieve the original clothes. It would have been less time consuming for all and more therapeutic for the patient had this seemingly simple request and activity been pursued both for the basic purpose of the activity itself as well as a cognitive/communicative treatment task.

The following are suggestions that will assist in turning routine unit tasks into a medium to help patients at this level of functioning to become cognitively organized:

1. Be calm and soothing in manner; move slowly, talk slowly and softly;
2. Present the patient with only one task at a time, and allow for completion of the entire task or a subpart of it before presenting the next task. Multiple tasks and instructions will only confuse the patient further;
3. Tell the patient what you want done several minutes before you actually start the task. Then tell the patient again just before you ask for an attempt of the task. This gives the patient time to become aware of you and the task and to begin to think about how to complete it. Sufficient time to process and organize the request and response is an essential part in helping the patient remain cognitively organized;
4. If the patient becomes confused and resists you and your request, do not continue the activity or begin talking. Wait until the patient appears relaxed and is attending to you and then explain the activity again and continue with it;
5. Give instructions at a time or in a place that is the most quiet and least distracting;
6. Before giving an instruction, be sure the patient is paying attention to you by placing yourself where you can be seen and then touch the patient before you begin talking;
7. Before giving an instruction, tell the patient what you want done and why it is needed to be done, then demonstrate what you want done and give the instruction;
8. When giving instructions, use gestures, demonstrations, and only a few of the most necessary and important words;
9. Once the sequence of routine unit activities has been established, do not change it and, whenever possible, do not change the personnel who carry the routine out. To the patient any such changes constitute a completely new task. The predictability of a routine is a major means of assisting the patient to remain cognitively organized.

Maintaining a structured environment is critical to patients at Levels V and VI. The environment includes the physical setting, the particular activity at hand, and the verbal and nonverbal interactions between the patient and others. The purpose of environmental structure is to keep the patient's environment as unconfusing as possible. If nursing activity is random, chaotic, and confusing, this will match and thereby indirectly reinforce the patient's own inner confusion.

Because patients at Levels V and VI are experiencing internal confusion, one of the best ways to treat the confusion is by modifying the environment to be less confusing. It is easier to modify the external confusion than to request patients to modify their internal confusion. An orderly, predictable, and structured environment will help patients remain at their highest level of function. The following are ways in which the environment can be modified to engender cognitive organization instead of precipitating disorganization.

1. Continue to employ suggestions 1 through 9 for level IV.
2. Describe the unit routine to the patient on a daily basis. This will help the patient understand why certain things are being done to and around him or her. Relate the description of the various unit routines to times of other unit events. In this way patients can gradually be helped to predict what is most likely to occur in their environment next by evaluating the present. The nurse can describe schedules for meals, medication, OT and PT, time to get up, time to go to bed, bathroom activities, visiting hours, and so on in relation to past and future events. For example: "It is 12 o'clock and you have finished lunch, next you will go to O.T." For unpredictable events or tasks, it will be helpful to describe these to the patient several times before you engage the patient in them. These might be such things as special appointments, rounds and conferences, special tests, any changes in the schedule, and so on.
3. Provide a constant verbal description of what the patient was doing, is doing, and what he or she is going to do. While it might be somewhat boring to the staff, verbal descriptions of what has occurred, is occurring, and will occur, will help the patient structure his or her behavior and relate it to things occurring in the environment;
4. Present all requests or instructions slowly and concisely. The patient should be given a few moments to think about what has been said before responding. Do not talk during these few moments, as the added speech will be confusing. If the patient does not respond appropriately, the request should be repeated. When it is repeated, attempt to use the same vocabulary and word order you originally used. Any slight change in either of these often causes the patient to think that you have made an entirely different request;
5. Keep the patient mentally challenged. Since CHI patients have difficulty structuring their environment, it will help if they are purposefully presented with structured tasks. Often if patients are allowed to remain

alone, they attend only to their fleeting and disjointed perceptions and thoughts. It is quite possible that this is one of the factors that eventually causes a patient to become agitated, combative, and even further confused.

Some of the things that might be done to challenge patients mentally during their free time are:

1. Encourage them to watch television;
2. Ask another patient to either talk with the CHI patient or go with them around the unit area and talk with people they meet;
3. Ask another patient or volunteer to read to them, play checkers or some similar game that will focus thoughts on a task.

Levels VII and VIII: Automatic-appropriate and purposeful-appropriate. The goal for this level is to assist the patient in carrying out daily unit routines with minimal to no supervision. One must be careful not to withdraw structured assistance too early with the Level VII patient. At this point the patient seems to look and act "normal" and, as a result, there is the tendency to assume he or she can carry out daily tasks in an appropriate manner. However, the appearance of normal functioning is only superficial. Underneath, the patient is still somewhat disorganized cognitively and retention span and short-term memory impairments are beginning to be visible as significant problems. While it may not appear so, the major reason the patient is able to function with the appearance of normalcy is because of the structure provided by the environment. If the structure is removed prematurely, the patient will begin to fluctuate between Level VI and VII. Consequently, the nursing approach should be one of continuing with the suggestions for Level VI but alternating the way in which they are used. Specifically, one should continue to supply the type of structure implicit in all of the suggestions given for Levels V and VI, but now only assist the patient to initiate the activity and help them with each task component. Now verbal instructions will not be needed several moments before a task and then repeated when it is initiated. However, it will still be important to present only one task and one instruction at a time. Providing structure and predictability of behavior through verbal descriptions can now be substantially decreased but not eliminated. Verbal structure should be used only for those activities or times where it is observed that the patient is becoming confused.

At this time, reduced retention span and short-term memory are beginning to emerge as the patients' more significant cognitive/communicative impairments. The nurse will find the following suggestions helpful in assisting the patient:

1. Have the patient's schedule located where it can be easily read by him or her. Be sure mornings and afternoons as well as the hours of the day are clearly marked and that the schedule is updated on a daily or hourly basis. The patient should be requested to refer to the schedule before and after each activity. If a staff member is with the patient, the patient should be encouraged to discuss what has just been completed and what is to be done next;

2. Have a clock and large calendar located in an easily visible place. Have the date of the given day indicated on the calendar. When patients are on the unit and away from their schedule, they should be asked to use the calendar and clock to determine what they are to do next in their routine. If they have difficulty, they should be asked to review their schedule. You should not give them the information. However, if they become confused, then you should go with the patients to the schedule board and review it with them until they are reoriented to what they are to do;

3. Patients in this phase of recovery are prone to become lost. This is a manifestation of the short-term memory problem. Because of this, it can be helpful to review with patients routes to and from activities. The patient should supply most of the information, with the nurse intervening only to supply correct information. It will be helpful to have a floor plan drawing available with such key areas as the patient's room, nursing station, and other treatment areas clearly marked. This can be used when patients have difficulty verbally describing a route. They can trace the path with their finger while simultaneously describing where they are expected to go;

4. Have patients keep a written daily log of their activities. Depending on each patient's length of short-term memory, the log may need to be filled out after each activity, at the end of a small block of time, or the end of the day.

GENERAL TREATMENT PRINCIPLES FOR ALL LEVELS OF COGNITIVE FUNCTIONING

The foregoing presented guidelines and suggestions as to how to stimulate, maintain, and enhance cognitive/communicative organization at each of the levels of cognitive functioning. There are, however, a number of general treatment principles that are applicable to all levels. The nurse can:

1. Keep the daily routine the same. It is extremely important to follow the same treatment routine and sequence of treatment tasks on a daily basis. The predictability of routine and tasks will considerably help the

patient's ability to cognitively organize responses. If the patient knows what is going to occur, he or she can plan for it. If the routine or tasks change frequently, CHI patients will then deal with the tasks as if each is completely new. This is the hardest thing for the patient to accomplish.

2. Use the patient's best channel of understanding. Stimuli should be presented through the patient's single most intact sensory modality (e.g. hearing, vision, touch, and so on) and increased to other modalities only as increasing cognitive abilities support the ability to deal with multiple stimuli.

3. Stimulate for and stabilize cognitive/communicative organization at the patient's most intact level of functioning. If treatment commences only at the level of deficit, the patient experiences a weakening of skills because of the increased cognitive demands. Under such conditions the patient then rapidly has two cognitive tasks; dealing with the original stimulus and simultaneously attempting to maintain the weakening subskills. By beginning with the lower level skills the patient is provided with the external structure that will be necessary to deal with the tasks that are at the level of dysfunction.

4. Present only one task at a time. Competing cognitive tasks force the patient to a lower level of functioning.

5. Manner of stimulus presentation is a critical factor. Present stimuli at a rate, amount, and duration that is consistent with the patient's best level of functioning at any moment. The manner of stimulus presentation is critical. If rate is too fast, amount too great, or duration too long, the patient will be forced to function at a lower level of behavior. It will be most helpful to keep daily information relative to these three variables with respect to the time of day and type of treatment. From this information one can derive a profile of how stimuli should be presented. However, because there will always be some fluctuations in the patient, those working with them should always be alert to behavioral cues that indicate the need to modify the manner of stimulus presentation.

Strategies for Management of the Communicative Dysfunction

Everything that a nurse does to, with, for, and around a patient will embody some form of communication with that patient. An understanding of the impact of the cognitive/communicative impairment upon patients and the manner in which they respond to their disorganized communication will be critical to the nurse's ability to develop a therapeutic environment.

The most observable aspect of the communication disorder is the patient's inability to either understand what others say and or to express words in a meaningful way. While the ability to use language is impaired, the disturbed language is not the impairment that affects the patient the most. The major impact of the communication disorder is that it blocks or impairs the patient's ability to either understand the needs, wants, thoughts, and feelings of others and or it impairs the patient's ability to enable another person to know his or her needs, wants, thoughts, and feelings. In essence the true impact of a communication disorder is not the inability to understand and or express words per se, but rather the effect that such impairments have on the individual's ability to interact with others socially, emotionally, and intellectually. The debilitating effect of a communication disorder is that it isolates patients from their surroundings. They are physically alive but in a state of suspended animation socially, emotionally, and intellectually. This state of isolation seriously erodes the patient's feelings of self-worth and interferes with the motivation to establish a new purpose in life—a reason for a "handicapped" person to continue living.

It is within this context that the nurse plays a significant role in the resolution of a patient's communication disorder. Typically, the nurse has more frequent contact with the patient than any other treating discipline; therefore, there are usually more communication attempts between the patient and nurse. The manner in which the nurse handles these attempts is a critical factor in helping patients remain in contact with their environment. The nurse's paramount goal for the communicatively impaired patient should be to prevent, limit, or delete the patient's feelings of isolation. There will be a direct relationship between the degree of isolation and the patient's communicative attempts. The more patients feel cut off from their surroundings the less they will attempt to communicate.

The more the nurse is successful in preventing feelings of isolation, the greater will be the patient's motivation to communicate. The patient's degree of motivation to communicate is quite critical to his or her ability to learn and use the communication skills that the speech-language pathologist is teaching.

The most effective means of preventing feelings of isolation, is to *communicate* with the patient. On the surface this may appear to be a very simplistic suggestion and might even be contrary to some of our natural impulses. For example, when confronted with an individual who is bleeding, our instinctive response is to stem the flow of blood. Similarly, when we encounter a communicatively impaired patient, our natural tendency is to teach them "words." We observe that the patient is struggling to say words and draw the logical conclusion that we can decrease the distress by teaching him or her to talk. However, patients' real sources of distress are the feelings that arise when they are unable to convey their inner needs, thoughts, and feelings to you. As such, emotional/social pain will be decreased to the degree to which they feel they have *communicated* with you, the degree to which they feel you *know* them at that moment.

Most assuredly, communication alone will not effectively alleviate a patient's specific speech and language disorder. However, the last thing patients need are well-meaning but unknowledgeable people trying to "teach words." Such attempts frequently lead to failure, the failure leads to frustration, and the frustration leads to either anger or depression. It is this emotional spiral that typically causes the patient to withdraw and feel isolated. A qualified speech-language pathologist should handle the direct treatment of the communication disorder. The following are suggestions of ways that a nurse can communicate with patients and thereby decrease their social, emotional, and intellectual isolation.

GENERAL SUGGESTIONS

1. Know your patient. Think a moment about your own typical daily household and work routine. Most probably you will find that the things you most frequently do are similar from day to day. Now think about your personal needs, wants, and concerns. These, too, probably remain somewhat the same across time. Finally, what do you most frequently need and or want to talk about? You may find considerable consistency from day to day here, too. In essence, the things we do, need, worry, and think about are, within limits, predictable. It is this predictability that allows individuals who know each other well to understand what each is saying without having to rely solely on the meaning of the words that are used. In a sense we need fewer words to communicate with those who know us well.

This same concept can be used by the nurse to establish a communication link with the patient. At the outset the nurse is at a distinct disadvantage. One does not know the patient well enough to be able to predict what the person is most probably attempting to communicate, and the patient cannot speak well enough to help the nurse know him or her. Under such circumstances one may very well include in the nursing treatment plan the goal of gathering enough pertinent information about a patient in order to *know* and, therefore, *communicate* with the patient. By increasing your familiarity with the patients, you will substantially increase your ability to predict what they are most probably attempting to communicate at a given time of the day, at a particular location in the hospital, and under certain surrounding circumstances.

Each individual is so multifaceted it would be impossible to know everything about a patient in a reasonable length of time. However, we have observed that a communicatively impaired patient in a hospital setting most frequently wants to communicate about something that falls within these categories:

(a) feelings (either the patient's feelings or the perception of others' feelings toward him or her);

(b) states of being (e.g. pain, need for food, warmth, fluid, or rest, concerns or questions about impaired body parts, and so on);

(c) people (family, friends, hospital personnel); and

(d) places (locations within or outside the hospital where the patient either has been or wishes to either go or not go).

The nurse will find it of considerable help in communicating with the patient if the patient's entire daily routine (day and night shift, on and off the ward) is thoroughly known. Observing the patient in respect to the four categories above and recording the observations in the patient's communication log relative to the individual's daily routine is essential to *knowing* your patient. Further, when a patient is attempting to communicate and the nurse eventually establishes what the message is, then both content and manner of communication is logged. At the end of 3 or 4 days the log should be reviewed and those items that have occurred most frequently identified. In most instances you will find that patients are no different than you are. They are usually fairly consistent in respect to which one or combination of the four categories they are attempting to communicate about. It will usually be a specific need, want, concern, and or opinion. Further, you will find that the manner in which they communicate the information remains the same.

2. Use alternate channels of communication. Under usual conditions the meaning of what we say is conveyed by the words we use, the way we say the words, and our general manner when speaking. In essence, communication relies on verbal as well as nonverbal behavior. The most typical nonverbal attributes of communication are (a) rate of speaking (e.g. a fast rate of speaking may signal excitement), (b) voice inflection (e.g. raising of pitch at the end of a sentence usually signals that the statement is a question, or unusually high or low pitch may signal extreme states of emotional distress), (c) loudness and emphasis of voice (e.g. sometimes signals a command or emphaticness of a statement), (d) the look in the individual's eyes, (e) facial expressions, (f) finger, hand, or arm gestures, and (g) overall body posture.

Most typically communicatively impaired patients continue to use nonverbal modes of communication just as they did before the injury. For this reason it is important to heighten your awareness and interpretation of a patient's nonverbal communication. To accomplish this when a patient is communicating, the nurse should pay specific attention to the voice, carefully watch eyes and face, and be aware of gestures and body postures that coincide with the communication attempts. Frequently the nurse will be able to quickly understand what the patient is communicating by correlating these nonverbal communications with knowledge of the patient gained from the communication log. At other times one may not be able to understand the specific content of a message, but if the nonverbal message has been understood, the nurse is still in a position of letting the patient know that the general feelings have been understood. While this result may not be totally satisfactory, patients will know that they have at least communicated a portion of their message.

Following are specific suggestions that can be useful when actually talking or listening to patients:

1. When talking to the patient:
   (a) Speak at a normal loudness level. Loud speech does not help the patient understand. On the contrary, it often confuses and upsets.
   (b) Speak at a slow rate of speech. Rapid speech confuses the patient and tends to block out what is heard. However, do not speak to the patient as if you are speaking to a kindergartner. This would be insulting to the adult patient.
   (c) Break up what you are saying into short sentences and allow a brief pause between each sentence. This will decrease confusion by allowing the patient to process small units of information completely.
   (d) When giving multiple instructions, give one at a time allowing the patient to respond to one instruction before proceeding to the next.
2. When the patient is talking to you:
   (a) Be sure you have the time to listen.
   (b) If you do—sit down, be calm and patient when you listen.
   (c) Use the communication log and your knowledge of patient's nonverbal communication characteristics to help you understand the content of the patient's message.
   (d) Do not try to supply a word which the patient is struggling to recall unless you are very sure you know what the word is.
   (e) Do not try to finish the patient's thought.
   (f) Do not interrupt or ask questions.
   (g) Ask questions when the patient stops.
   (h) Do not tell the patient you understand if you don't.
3. When patients cannot understand spoken speech, visual demonstrations, pictures, or words, then they should be approached only through physical demonstrations as described previously.

CONCLUSIONS

Some of the general ideas and specific suggestions put forth in this chapter may appear very time-consuming. In fact, they are when compared with normal communication processes or communicative interactions with non-brain-injured patients. With the prevailing high patient-to-staff ratios, time utilization is a primary concern to all health care disciplines. Most certainly the nurse must take into consideration the needs of all of the patients on the unit and prioritize time accordingly. However, in my experience, cognitive/communicative disorganized patients are less time-consuming when the nurse is able to communicate with them and maintain their highest level of cognitive organization. Under such circumstances, patients understand what they are to do and proceed as independently as possible. Consequently, not only will a therapeutic nursing unit environment decrease the amount of nursing time with the patient, but it will also have a significant positive impact on the patient's overall rehabilitation.

REFERENCES

Adams, R., & Sidmann, R.L. *Introduction to neuropathology.* New York: McGraw-Hill, 1968.

Brain, W.R., & Walton, J.N. *Brain's diseases of the nervous system*, (7th ed.) London: Oxford University Press, 1969.

Courville, C.B. Coup, contre-coup mechanisms of craniocerebral injuries: Some observations. *Archives of Surgery*, 1942, *45*, 19–43.

Courville, C.B., & Amyes, E.W. Late residual lesions of the brain consequent to dural hemorrhage. *Bulletin Los Angeles Neurology Society*, 1952, *17*, 163.

Cronholm, B. Evaluation of mental disturbances after acute head injury. *Scandinavian Journal of Rehabilitation Medicine*, 1972, *4*, 35–38.

Dye, O.A., Milby, J.B., & Saxon, S.A. Effects of early neurological problems following head trauma on subsequent neurological performance. *Acta Neurologic Scandinavia*, 1979, *59*, 10–14.

Feild, J.R. Head injuries pathophysiology. *Journal Arkansas Medical Association*, 1970, *66*, 340–347.

Greenfield, J.G. Some observations on cerebral injuries. *Proceedings Royal Society of Medicine*, 1938–39, *32*, 45.

Greenfield, J.G., & Russell, D.S. Traumatic lesions of the central and peripheral nervous systems. In W. Blackwood (Ed.), *Greenfield's neuropathology.* Chicago: Year Book, 1963.

Hagen, C., & Malkmus, D. *Intervention strategies for language disorders secondary to head trauma.* American Speech-Language-Hearing Association Convention Short Course, Atlanta, 1979.

Hooper, R. *Patterns of acute head injury.* Baltimore: Williams & Wilkins, 1969.

Horowitz, N., & Rizzoli, H.V. *Complications following the surgical treatment of head injuries, clinical neurosurgery,* Proceedings of the Congress of Neurological Surgeons, 1966, 277–287.

Jacobson, S.A. Disturbances of mental function—Effects of head trauma on mental function. In S.A. Jacobson (Ed.), *Post traumatic syndrome following head injury—Mechanisms and treatment.* Springfield, IL: Charles C. Thomas, 1963.

Jennett, B., & Teasdale, G. Aspects of coma after severe head injury. *Lancet,* 1977, (2), 878–881.

Jennett, B., & Teasdale, G. *Management of head injuries.* Philadelphia: F.A. Davis Co., 1981.

Lewin, W. *The management of head injuries.* Baltimore: Williams & Wilkins, 1966.

Mandleberg, I.A., & Brooks, D.N. Cognitive recovery after severe head injury. *Journal of Neurology, Neurosurgery and Psychiatry,* 1975, *38,* 1121–1126.

Meyer, J.S., & Denny-Brown, D. Studies of cerebral circulation in brain injury. II. Cerebral concussion. *Neurophysiology,* 1955, *7,* 529–544.

Rowbotham, G.F. *Acute injuries of the head* (4th ed.).Edinburgh: E. & S. Livingstone, Ltd., 1964.

Russell, R.W. Cerebral involvement in head injury. *Brain,* 1932, *55,* 549–603.

Schilder, P. Psychic disturbance after head injuries. *American Journal of Psychiatry,* 1934, *91,* 155–188.

Strich, S.J. Diffuse degeneration of the cerebral white matter in severe dementia following head injury. *Journal of Neurology and Psychiatry,* 1956, *19,* 163.

Teasdale, G., & Jennett, B. Assessment of coma and impaired consciousness: A practical scale. *Lancet,* 1974 (2), 81–84.

Tomlinson, B.E. Pathology. In G.F. Rowbotham (Ed.), *Acute injuries of the head* (4th ed.). Edinburgh: E. & S. Livingstone, Ltd., 1964.

Walker, A.E., Kabros, J.J., & Case, T.J. The physiological basis of concussion. *Journal Neurosurgery,* 1944, *1,* 103–116.

7

Retraining Swallowing
After Brain Injury

Barbara E. Aliza

INTRODUCTION

Difficulty in swallowing, or *dysphagia*, in the brain injured patient has long been recognized as a significant clinical problem. Dysphagia is frequently associated with a number of disorders commonly seen in acute care and rehabilitation settings (Table 7-1). In addition to being present in neuromuscular disorders, dysphagia is also seen as a result of local structural lesions and radiation therapy, and as a result of disorders affecting normal motor development. It may also have a strong psychogenic component.

For information specific to head and neck cancer and developmental swallowing problems, see Fust (1973) and Gallender (1979), respectively.

The impact of a swallowing problem on the psychological as well as the physical well being of the patient cannot be overlooked. Imagine, for example, what it must be like to awake within minutes, hours, or perhaps days of some neurological trauma and discover that you cannot perform some of the most simple, basic functions you were previously able to do without thought. In the process of taking stock of yourself, you find you are unable to move your arm; your leg seems paralyzed. People are talking to you and you can't

TABLE 7-1

Specific disorders associated with dysphagia

Neuromuscular Lesions	*Local Structural Lesions*
Cerebral vascular accident (CVA)	Surgical resection of oropharynx
Parkinson's disease	Oropharyngeal carcinoma
Huntington's chorea	(e.g., glossectomy)
Amyotrophic lateral	Laryngeal cancer
sclerosis (ALS)	Inflammation disorders
Encephalitis	Diverticulum
Meningitis	Webs—hypopharyngeal and
Anoxia	esophageal
Demyelinating diseases	Plummer Vinson syndrome
(e.g., Multiple sclerosis)	Extrinsic compression
Head trauma	retropharyngeal abscess
Tabes dorsalis	thyroid enlargement
Brain stem tumors	senile ankylosing hyperostosis
Changes associated with	of cervical spine
advancing age	enlarged lymph nodes
Changes associated with	
radiation therapy	
Miscellaneous congenital and or	
degenerative disorders	
Syringomyelia	
Bulbar poliomyelitis	
Peripheral neuropathy	
(e.g., diabetes, alcoholism)	
Myasthenia gravis	
Inflammatory muscle disease	
Muscular dystrophies	
Metabolic myopathy	

make sense out of what they are saying. You try to talk, but no one seems to understand. Breathing may be difficult—perhaps you are on a respirator or receiving oxygen. As you struggle to swallow, you begin to cough or choke—the saliva in your mouth threatens to overwhelm you. There is a hard tube in your throat and nose and liquid is slowly dripping through the tube into your stomach.

As health professionals who experience intense daily contact with patients, it is not difficult for us to imagine ourselves in this situation. We may also be able to call on our common experiences of almost choking on a piece of food or of briefly panicking when it was difficult to swallow with a severe sore throat. Whether the onset of a swallowing problem is sudden or the result of a slow degenerative process, the physical and psychological effects are serious. The brain-injured patient who experiences dysphagia is concerned with survival. How can life be sustained without swallowing? The fear of choking, of not being able to eat or drink, or of having to depend on being fed with a tube for the remainder of life, can be overwhelming.

Potential Pathological Problems

In addition to psychological trauma, the potential physical difficulties the brain-injured patient can experience secondary to swallowing dysfunction are numerous and complex. They include:

1. Inadequate nourishment
2. Diarrhea due to a tube fed liquid diet
3. Aspiration and aspiration pneumonia
4. Irritation of mucous membranes in the nose, pharynx, esophagus, and stomach from the nasogastric (NG) tube, with potential for ulceration
5. Decreased sensation in the pharynx due to the presence of NG tube
6. Esophageal reflux
7. Infection from surgically inserted tubes
8. If tracheostomy tube is present, then: decreased sensation in trachea and reduced frequency of reflexive swallow, excessive pressure on walls of trachea and esophagus with potential for fistulas, and interference with the normal excursion of the laryngeal mechanism during swallowing
9. Development of improper swallowing patterns as well as repetitive and self-stimulating oral movement
10. Associated problems with speech function

(Aliza, 1979, 1980; Burke, 1978; Griffin, 1974; Roueche, 1980)

Intervention and the Team Approach

The potential for the aforementioned pathological problems underscores the need to evaluate the procedures traditionally employed and to look at the new and successful therapy techniques offered by a team of health professionals with very specific expertise.

Traditionally, the approach to swallowing dysfunction has been to "wait and see" what will happen neurologically and to effectively bypass the active swallow, with intervention limited to tube feeding (Aliza, 1979, 1980; Burke, 1978). Although there are a variety of tube feedings that have been utilized, the nasogastric tube has been most commonly employed as the immediate and temporary solution. On a long-term basis, the gastrostomy has been popular if the patient was able to tolerate the surgical procedure. Rehabilitative surgery has also been utilized, but success has been limited to very specific types of impairment. Common examples of compensatory surgeries are the teflon injection and the crico-pharyngeal myotomy (Dobie, 1978). The teflon injection into the paralyzed vocal fold allows the folds to close the airway more tightly, thus protecting the airway from intrusion by foods or liquids. A crico-pharyngeal myotomy opens the esophagus to food when there is spasticity present in the musculature.

For further information on gastrostomies, see Brunner and Suddarth (1978).

A review of the literature reveals that in the last 10 years there have been significant contributions to the active retraining of the swallow by nurses, speech-language pathologists, occupational and physical therapists, and physicians (Buckley, Addicks, & Maniglia, 1976; Gaffney & Campbell, 1974; Hargrove, 1980; Larsen, 1973; Robins, Adkins, Linquist, Lim, & Dail, 1958; Seaman, 1976). Only recently, however, have a number of consistent and effective therapy programs begun to emerge which utilize the expertise of a variety of health professionals in a coordinated team approach. Knowledge about positioning, reflexes, type and texture of food, nutritional and medical needs, neurophysiological factors, oral facial motor function, cognitive and language needs, and social/environmental factors is being recognized as essential for assessment and treatment of the dysphagic patient (Aliza, 1979, 1980; Burke, 1978; Roueche, 1980; Winstein, 1980). A variety of facilitative techniques has been gathered and developed which offer viable alternatives to the traditional approaches.

THE NORMAL SWALLOW

Before discussing management of the dysphagic patient, let us analyze the normal swallowing process. A clear understanding of this process is necessary to acquire a rationale for intervention.

The act of swallowing, or deglutition, is a complex neuromuscular act requiring the coordinated action of multiple structures (Hurwitz, Nelson, &

Haddad, 1975) (See Figure 7–1) and involving over 20 muscle pairs (Johnson & Johnson, 1976). Swallowing occurs quickly and continuously, normally completing its action in 5 to 7 seconds (Dobie, 1978) at an average of twice a minute when not eating. Although the orderly participation of the multiple structures involved is controlled, in large part by the brain stem, the cortex also has significant influence on both a sensory and motor level (Gray, 1973). This influence will become clearer as our discussion continues.

The purpose of swallowing is to transport food, liquid, and saliva from the mouth through the pharynx and the esophagus into the stomach. The process is commonly discussed as occurring in three phases: *oral, pharyngeal,* and *esophageal* (Dobie, 1978; Fust, 1973) corresponding to the three cavities through which the food and liquid travel on the way to the stomach. (See Figure 7–2.)

Oral Phase

After chewing is completed, the oral phase is quite rapid, lasting from .3 to 1 second (Dobie, 1978). Cranial nerves V, VII, and XII (see Figure 7–3) participate in this phase (Dobie, 1978) by innervating the muscles which receive the food, chew it, and move it to the pharynx. The oral phase begins when the food is placed in the mouth and is picked up by the tongue and proceeds as follows:

1. Jaw closes, lips together and relaxed
2. Muscles of the palate, tongue, and cheeks form the food into a bolus; sucking action helps to center it on the tongue (see Figure 7–2, b)
3. Tongue tip contacts the alveolar ridge, remaining there while the entire tongue lifts upward along with a slight upward movement of the larynx; the sucking and lifting action of the tongue moves the food backwards (see Figure 7–2, c)
4. The pharyngeal portion of the tongue arches up behind the bolus while the soft palate contracts downward and the faucial pillars contract towards midline
5. Tongue tip and sides remain fixed against the ridge and teeth, respectively

(Dobie, 1978; Gray, 1973; Larsen, 1973)

The interaction between the cortex and the brain stem during this phase is significant. Salivation is necessary for swallowing to occur, and it is stimulated by the sight, smell, and palatability of food—all cortical functions. Decisions as to what we like or don't like in foods and what we will accept or reject are made at this level also. Although chewing can be reflexive, it too can be controlled by the cortex and can be stopped, accelerated, or slowed down at will.

FIGURE 7–1
Multiple structures involved in swallowing

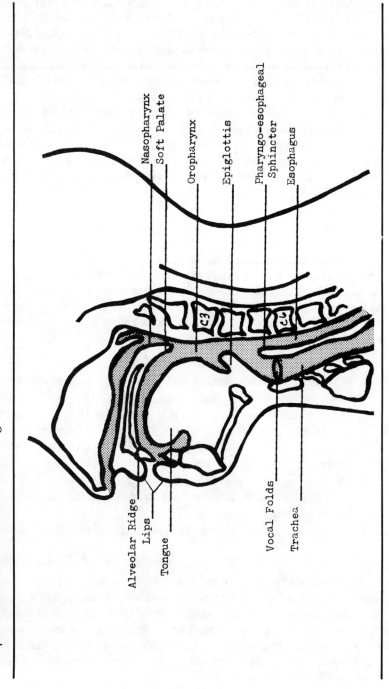

FIGURE 7-2
Sequence of the normal swallow

NOTE: From "Rehabilitation of Swallowing Disorders" by R.A. Dobie, *American Family Physician*, 1978, *17*, 84–94. Copyright 1978 by American Family Physician. Reprinted by permission.

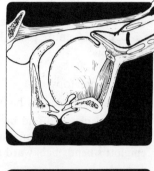

a. Mouth and pharynx at rest

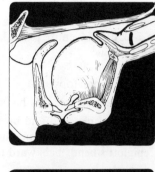

b. Early oral phase

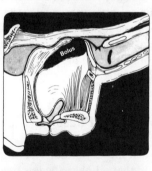

c. Late oral phase

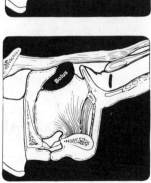

d. Early pharyngeal phase

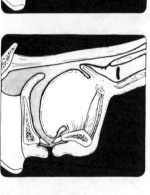

e. Middle pharyngeal phase

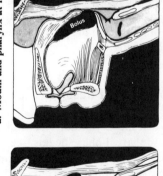

f. Late pharyngeal phase

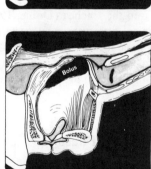

g. Esophageal phase

Pharyngeal Phase

When the base of the tongue lowers, allowing the food to enter the oropharynx and stimulate its receptors, the pharyngeal phase begins (see Figure 7–2, d). The entire phase lasts only one second, following the course described below:

1. Respiration stops
2. Soft palate closes off the nasopharynx as the oropharynx contracts
3. Larynx is elevated and brought forward; upper esophageal sphincter relaxes while, simultaneously, the vocal folds approximate and the epiglottis bends backward to form a chute over the larynx (see Figure 7–2, e)
4. The base of the tongue pushes against the posterior wall of the pharynx and this is followed by a contraction of the pharyngeal constrictors, resulting in a wave of motion that empties the pharynx (see Figure 7–2, f)

(Dobie, 1978; Gray, 1973; Larsen, 1973)

It is the upward and forward motion of the larynx that is most important in protecting the airway; the epiglottis is relatively unimportant. The closure of the vocal folds acts as the second line of defense in preventing leakage of food into the trachea (Dobie, 1978; Zemlin, 1968).

Clinical observation suggests that although this phase cannot be terminated once it has begun, cortical control can be exerted over its functions. Patients appear able to consciously maintain and even increase the contraction of muscles of the pharynx and vocal folds. This phase can also be slowed or accelerated to some extent.

Esophageal Phase

When the larynx descends and the upper esophageal sphincter contracts, the esophageal phase begins (see Figure 7–2, g). This phase lasts from 3 to 7 seconds (Dobie, 1978). Respiration begins and food travels down the esophagus by peristaltic action (Larsen, 1973). The lower esophageal sphincter must relax to allow the food to enter the stomach and then close to avoid reflux.

THE ABNORMAL SWALLOW (DYSPHAGIA)

The multiple structures involved in swallowing must work in a coordinated manner for swallowing to be efficient and safe. Any difficulty or dysfunction in any one of the phases just discussed is referred to as dysphagia. It is common to see problems in both the oral and pharyngeal phases simultaneously, although you may also see just one phase affected. The retraining of swallowing function is very useful with problems in the oral and pharyngeal phases, but is not appropriate for esophageal phase problems.

Oral Phase Problems

When there is facial and oral muscle weakness or dysfunction, the patient may well have problems with the oral phase (Dobie, 1978). Problems in this area are characterized by one or more of the following: drooling, oral retention of food, leakage of liquids from the mouth, and insufficiently chewed food (Aliza, 1980; Roueche, 1980). The patient may also demonstrate abnormal head posture during eating (Roueche, 1980) that reflects an attempt to move the food back into the throat. Also noted in the oral phase may be difficulty in initiating and following through with the swallow pattern (Larsen, 1972).

Pharyngeal Phase Problems

When there is poor palatal closure, impairment of the muscles in the pharyngeal wall, poor epiglottic function, inadequate vocal fold closure and or inadequate elevation of the pharynx and larynx during the swallow, and or spasticity of the pharyngo-esophageal sphincter, there is a pharyngeal phase problem. Symptoms include: nasal regurgitation of food because the nasopharynx has not been sealed off by action of the soft palate; coughing, choking, and or aspiration of swallowed material; or incomplete passage of food through the pharyngo-esophageal sphincter and retention of food in the pharynx and piriform sinuses (Aliza, 1980; Roueche, 1980). The latter two symptoms are evidenced by a delay in aspiration of 5 to 7 seconds after swallowing and or the coughing up of food after swallowing. This problem suggests spasticity in the pharyngo-esophageal sphincter and requires further assessment by an otolaryngologist and radiologist.

Esophageal Phase Problems

If there is reflux of swallowed material or if the patient complains of fullness or of the food getting "stuck" in the esophageal area, then an esophageal phase problem should be suspected. These symptoms suggest a dysfunction of the lower esophageal sphincter or some obstruction in the esophageal tube. Frequently, the patient can correctly identify the site of the problem (Seaman, 1976).

FIGURE 7-3
Cranial nerves involved in swallowing

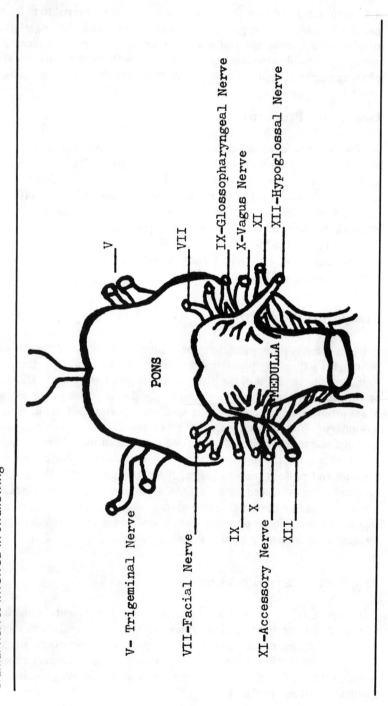

CAUSES OF DYSPHAGIA

Although Table 7-1 provided us with a fairly complete outline of the various specific disorders that may have dysphagia as a component, we need to look at why these disorders affect swallowing function in the brain-injured patient. As we stated previously, swallowing is controlled by both the brain stem and the cortex. Therefore, we are concerned with dysphagia that can occur as a result of lesions in certain cranial nerves, their nuclei or fiber tracts, or as a result of injury to the cortex. Because of differences in symptomatology, it is best to discuss etiology with respect to classification as either *bulbar palsy*, a lower motor neuron lesion, or *pseudo-bulbar palsy*, an upper motor neuron lesion. Lesions of either type can cause problems in one or more of the three phases of swallowing.

Bulbar Palsy: A Lower Motor Neuron Lesion

The brain stem is the part of the brain which connects the spinal cord with the cerebrum. The medulla oblongata of the brain stem, see Figure 7-3, or bulb, as it is called, is referred to as the swallowing center (Gray, 1973). The cranial nerves involved in swallowing, V, VII, IX, X, XI, and XII, either arise from the medulla or synapse there and then directly supply specific muscles—those of the lips, tongue, jaw, palate, pharynx, larynx, and esophagus. Because of their direct route to the muscles of swallowing, these cranial nerves, their nuclei, and fiber tracts, along with the first three cervical nerve segments which communicate specifically with cranial nerves X, XI, and XII, are considered lower motor neurons. Any impairment, therefore, at the level of the medulla (or bulb) is referred to as *bulbar palsy*.

Specific symptoms of this type of lesion include paralysis of individual muscles and or weakness or flaccidity. There will be weakness of muscle contraction, hypotonia, loss of muscle stretch reflexes, muscle atrophy, and fasciculations (Darley, Aronson, & Brown, 1975).

Pseudo-Bulbar Palsy: An Upper Motor Neuron Lesion

Impairment at any level above the medulla and in the cortex is referred to as pseudo-bulbar palsy. The symptomatology mirrors that of bulbar palsy in that there is weakness, but also differs (Darley et al., 1975; Larsen, 1973). Lesions can occur in either the sensory or motor strip of the cortex where specific areas are responsible for the specific motor functions linked to the cranial nerves in the swallowing process. Lesions, however, must be bilateral in the cortex to effect permanent impairment (Darley et al., 1975). Dysphagia, resulting from a unilateral cortical lesion, would resolve very quickly due to the significant crossover of function at the cortical level.

Symptoms of pseudo-bulbar palsy include muscle weakness, as in bulbar palsy, and spasticity and impairment in movement patterns (Darley et al., 1975). One easily distinguishable feature with respect to dysphagia is the difficulty in initiating the act of swallowing and in maintaining it to completion. There is also incoordination of movement patterns required for swallowing. Spasticity can extend as far as the diaphragm but is not readily observable. There is no atrophy of musculature; abnormal reflexes may be present; tongue movements tend to be slow; and impairment in affect may well be present (Darley et al., 1975).

MANAGEMENT

Successful management begins with a thorough evaluation of the swallowing problem. The utilization of the expertise of a number of health professionals in assessing the problem will ensure that all factors have been considered. It is one thing to know what phase of the swallowing is impaired, but do we know how certain reflexes might exacerbate the problem and how to inhibit those reflexes? Do we know if we can change the tracheostomy tube to effect greater laryngeal movement? Perhaps there are respiratory problems which preclude the use of milk products in the feeding. Some medical problems may require additional nutritional intake or there may be a need for further assessment through radiology.

These questions can best be answered when the rehabilitation team approaches the problem in a coordinated way. A discussion of the specific responsibilities of each team member will provide a clear outline of the factors that need to be evaluated on an ongoing basis. We will then discuss specific evaluation and treatment considerations accumulated through the direct clinical experience of this author as well as through the reported experience of a number of clinical programs (Aliza, 1980; Burke, 1978; Griffin, 1974; Larsen, 1973; Roueche, 1980; St. Jude's Hospital, 1981; Winstein, 1980).

The Rehabilitation Team

The nurse is frequently the person who first recognizes the presence of swallowing difficulty and initiates a referral to the team. The assessment of dysfunction, the design of treatment, and the coordination of the team is usually carried out by the speech-language pathologist and or the occupational therapist, although this varies from setting to setting. Specific responsibilities of each member include:

> *The nurse:* provides a history of patient's eating habits, onset of problem, details regarding the current method of food intake and tracheostomy care, type and size of tracheostomy and nasogastric tubes, and information about diet and medical concerns affecting treatment. Direct nursing care includes suctioning and tracheostomy care assistance and the implementation of the training program at all meals when an adequate swallow has been established. The nurse may also assist in training the family. Records regarding caloric count, intake and output, and the presence or absence of aspiration are kept. Medications are given in a manner consistent with the swallowing progam.

> *The speech-language pathologist:* obtains appropriate background information from the nurse, family, and physician and directly evaluates oral-facial and swallowing function, cognitive function, and communication needs. Treatment is designed with respect to diet, positioning, environmental considerations, and the use of specific facilitation techniques. After initiating the treatment program, the speech-language pathologist trains the nursing staff and occupational therapist in carrying over the progam and assists in training the family. Ongoing supervision of the program is maintained.

> *The occupational and physical therapists:* assist the presence or absence of specific reflexes which may affect swallowing function. Recommendations are made on positioning the patient for proper head control and body righting needs during feeding and on ways to inhibit or facilitate motor function. The occupational therapist contributes to cognitive assessment and, when appropriate, begins to train patients to feed themselves.

> *The dietician:* determines a special diet based on information from nursing and speech-language pathology and monitors fluid and caloric intake.

> *The respiratory therapist:* although involvement varies in each setting, provides important information regarding respiratory function, the type of tracheostomy apparatus to be used, the patient's ability to cough and clear the airway, and the necessary precautions around tracheostomy care and feeding. Assistance may also be given in suctioning and in monitoring of aspiration.

> *The social worker:* provides information regarding the patient, family, and the environment to which the patient will be discharged.

This is necessary to establish realistic goals and procedures.

The physician: authorizes referral to the team and contributes information regarding etiology and ongoing status of the patient. Consultation regarding further assessment and medical treatment is given.

The dysphagia team can function on either a formal or informal basis. Of paramount importance is that as the patient progresses in the program there is ongoing communication between team members. Nurses play an integral part in the treatment program due to their nursing and medical expertise, their consistent contact with the patient, physician, and family, and their responsibilities for coordination of the overall care of the patient.

Assessment Considerations

Prior to direct evaluation of oral-facial and swallowing function important background information is gathered by the evaluator, usually the speech-language pathologist. This information is helpful in preparing for direct assessment. For example, knowledge of whether the patient has a bulbar palsy or a pseudo-bulbar palsy will provide clues as to the functional nature of the problem—especially when it may not be readily observed, as in the case of spasticity. The nasogastric tube may need to be changed prior to evaluation or even removed. The tube, itself, should not be larger than a #12 so as to minimize interference with sensory function in the pharynx and esophagus; the longer it is in place the more likely its affect on sensation. A tracheostomy button or Jackson trach, size 4 or smaller, should be used if possible to minimize its interference with laryngeal excursion (Johnson & Johnson, 1976). Care should be taken to present test foods that correspond to the patient's preferences. Knowledge of current means of food intake and diet restrictions is also important.

Direct evaluation involves assessment of oral-facial and swallowing function. The evaluator must look for specific muscle weakness or incoordination of the lips, tongue, palate, pharynx, jaw, and vocal folds. The intactness of the gag reflex is assessed along with symmetry of movement and sensation of the oral structures. The cough and swallow must be evaluated on both a spontaneous and voluntary level. One needs to determine if the swallow can be stimulated and how. How well does the patient handle secretions? Do different tastes, textures, and viscosities affect the swallowing process? Is there evidence of poor coordination of the three phases?

For specific techniques in conducting an oral-facial peripheral exam, see Emerick and Hatten (1974).

After determination is made as to which phase or phases of the swallow are involved and to what extent, recommendations are made as to diet, environmental controls, the need for assistance from nursing or respiratory therapy during the training sessions, specific positioning requirements, and specific facilitation techniques. Identification of goals should be made with consideration given to prognosis and to where the patient will be discharged, so that a realistic program can be designed.[1] The patient may be going home or to an extended care facility. The team needs to know that if ongoing supervision of swallowing is needed, those responsible for the supervision are capable of following through.

Treatment Considerations

There are a number of variables which must be considered in establishing a program for retraining swallowing in the brain-injured adult. Because we are dealing with neurologically impaired patients, each patient will demonstrate a number of problems and symptoms—some which are unique to the patient and some which are consistent among all dysphagic patients. For these reasons each patient must be considered individually. A treatment program is established and refined on an ongoing basis. Once an effective and consistent swallow is established with minimum danger of aspiration, responsibility for carrying out the program at all meals is transferred to the nursing staff. Specific directions and demonstration should be provided for the nurse while supervision of the program will be maintained by the speech-language pathologist. As the patient progresses, the nurse may have to modify the program in consultation with the team.

Specific considerations for treatment include:

Environment. Controlling the environment in which therapy is taking place is essential in maximizing the patient's conscious control over the swallowing process. It is common for neurologically impaired patients to demonstrate reduced attention span and to have difficulty relating appropriately to people and objects around them. Therefore, it is essential for the environment to be free of distractions such as television, ongoing tube feedings, and extraneous people, conversations, and objects.

The environment must be simple with a minimum of verbalizations. The patient should be as comfortable as possible. It is helpful to schedule oral feedings before a tube feeding so that the patient is hungry. Placing food near the patient's bed a few minutes prior to feeding, so that it can be seen and smelled, is effective in stimulating the production of saliva.

Positioning. Maximal protection of the airway can be achieved by positioning the patient in a 90° sitting position with hips flexed, shoulders relaxed and slightly rounded, and the head flexed slightly forward. This position places the larynx further under the base of the tongue and, therefore, under its protection from intrusion of swallowed material into the larynx. Although this may not offer complete protection, it is frequently all that is needed to effect a safe swallow. If trunk control is poor, support may be given by pillows. Additional suggestions for positioning may be given by the physical or occupational therapist. The suggestions will be specific to the individual patient and may assist in inhibiting certain reflexes. When positioned, the patient's head should be facing forward—not tilted to either side—to avoid pooling of food. The person feeding the patient should be sitting at the level of the patient and in front so that positioning is maintained. Medications should be given in a similar manner. Swallowing therapy should not be attempted if positioning cannot be controlled.

Diet. Control of the diet is another essential element in maximizing protection of the airway and in stimulating a more normal process. Temperatures, textures, tastes, and viscosities can be manipulated, but it is important to try to utilize foods in natural forms if possible so attractiveness, taste, and ability to stimulate receptors are maintained. Care should be taken that foods are not too hot or too cold, but slightly warmer or colder than body temperature. The variance from body temperature will enhance stimulation.

The appropriate diet level (Table 7–2) should be determined in the evaluation session by having available a variety of tastes and textures and progressing from the easiest to the more difficult as the patient demonstrates an ability to handle foods. It is strongly recommended that water or any other thin liquid not be given to the patient if there is evidence of aspiration with foods at Stage I of the dysphagia diet. Liquids, water in particular, are characteristically the most difficult to swallow because they move quickly with gravity, requiring precise coordination of muscle movement. Solid foods move with peristaltic action and, therefore, more slowly.

Stage I of the diet consists of foods that pass easily through the mouth and pharynx and can be placed precisely in the mouth and easily suctioned if aspiration occurs. Periodically, food should be colored with blue vegetable dye so that any presence of food in the trachea can be easily determined on suctioning. If, after the patient swallows, there is a delay of 5 to 7 seconds before coughing begins and if the patient coughs up some of the food just swallowed, then the pharyngo-esophageal sphincter may be in spasm and not allowing the food to pass into the esophagus. In this case, the swallowing of liquids should be assessed. Frequently, patients with spasticity in this area can handle liquids, but not solids.

If the nurse or respiratory therapist determines the presence of a respiratory problem, then milk products should be avoided to prevent thickening of secretions. The dietician can offer alternatives.

TABLE 7-2

Diet guidelines for a dysphagic patient

Solids		
	Stage 1:	Yogurt[1]
		Applesauce
		Smooth hot cereals (e.g.: Cream of Wheat, blended oatmeal)
		Puddings
		Custard (broken up)
		Jello (chopped up)
		Bananas (well-mashed, pureed)
		Avocado (well-mashed)
		Pureed fruit
		Ice cream/sherbet
	Stage 2:	All of the above
		Soft-boiled or poached egg (very moist)
		Loosely scrambled eggs
		Oatmeal (moistened with milk)
		Cottage cheese (loose and moist)
		Mashed bananas (lumpy)
		Finely chopped canned fruit (peaches, pears, apricots)
		Pureed meats (lumpy and moistened, if necessary[2])
		Mashed avocado (lumpy)
		Pureed or mashed cooked vegetables (peas, carrots, squash—nothing stringy)
		Mashed potatoes (moistened)
	Stage 3:	All of the above
		Toast (without crust and moistened; broken into small pieces)
		Canned fruit (chopped)
		Bananas (chopped or sliced)
		Finely ground meats (moistened)
		Baked fish (no bones)
		Chopped cooked vegetables
		Egg salad (moistened)
		Pasta or rice
		Macaroni salad

TABLE 7-2 (continued)

	Stage 4:	All of the above Coarsely ground meat (like ground beef) Well-baked chicken Coarsely chopped cooked vegetables Chopped fresh tomatoes Coarsely chopped salad
Liquids	**Stage 1:**	Thick milk shakes Thick tomato juice or fruit juice Juice thickened with gelatin
	Stage 2:	Liquids of normal viscosity Carbonated drinks
Minimum Requirements	Liquids: Calories:	1500 cc's—Adult 900 cc's—Child Determined by weight
Equivalents	Liquids: Solids:	1 oz. equals 30 cc's 30 oz. equals 900 cc's 4 one cup servings equals 900 cc's Jello is considered to be a clear liquid Some of the liquid intake is drawn from the liquid content of solid foods.

This diet prepared by:
Barbara Aliza, MA, CCC
Speech-Language Pathologist

[1]Milk products should not be given if excess secretions are a problem

[2]Moistening of certain foods can be achieved with meat or vegetable stock

Pre-feeding stimulation techniques. Prior to the introduction of food in a treatment session, it is very important to stimulate salivation, a swallow, and oral-motor function in general. A variety of oral-motor exercises and stimulation techniques can be utilized in combination to accomplish this (Langley & Darvill, 1979):

(1) Use of resistive and range of motion exercises for the tongue and lips

(2) Brushing and icing of the lips, cheeks, and external laryngeal area in a prescribed manner to facilitate motor function (It is important that an occupational therapist be consulted before utilizing this technique, as specific training is needed.)

(3) Use of a lemon glycerine swab in a backward and forward motion on the tongue to stimulate saliva production and therefore sucking and swallowing

(4) Touching the soft palate or faucial pillars with a tongue blade or swab to stimulate a gag reflex; this is an important reflex for protection of the airway

(5) Closing of the mouth and pulling the jaw slightly forward to allow collected saliva to fall back into the pharynx and thus stimulate a swallow

(6) Walking backward on the tongue at midline with a tongue blade to stimulate a swallow

(7) Rocking the laryngeal mechanism laterally as the patient is talked through a swallow

(8) Helping patients to visualize muscle contraction as they think through the swallow

These techniques are just a few of the facilitation techniques available to the speech-language pathologist. Their importance lies in strengthening musculature, increasing range of motion, and focusing the patient's attention on oral movements involved in swallowing. Although these should be an essential part of each treatment session, failure of the patient to effect a swallow or to participate in exercises does not necessarily preclude the introduction of food. The patient may be severely apraxic[2] and may respond more effectively with food. The decision to present food must be made by an experienced speech-language pathologist with safeguards ready in case of aspiration.

For additional information on facilitation techniques, see Gallender (1979); Mysak (1973); Roueche (1980); St. Jude's Hospital (1981).

Facilitation techniques with feeding. Before feeding begins make sure
the patient's mouth is clean so that taste can be maximized. Check positioning and environmental factors. Then choose the implements that will
allow the greatest control. A 60cc catheter tip syringe will allow accurate
placement of food on the tongue. Placement of food will be posterior if
patient has difficulty moving it backwards and lateralized if sensation is
more intact on one side. If optimum placement is lateral, care should be
taken to place food as close to midline as possible. The use of a syringe
requires careful attention to: 1). maintaining the proper positioning of the
patient, 2). to the injection of no more than 3cc's of liquid at a time, and
3). to accurate placement of the liquid so that the patient can control its
movement. The use of a spoon requires patients to close their mouths
around it, which is part of the swallowing pattern. The problem, however,
is that the spoon requires patients to move the food back on their own.
Depressing the spoon on the middle of the tongue and then quickly pulling
the spoon up and out also stimulates a correct swallowing pattern. The
use of a cup with liquids is difficult because many patients cannot control
the amount they take in at one time and also have trouble closing their
mouths around the edge. A syringe or straw can be used to place liquids
precisely.

Only small bites or sips should be taken and each should be swallowed
completely before the next is given. If, after the food is placed, patients have
difficulty initiating or completing the swallow, help them to close their
mouths and talk them through the swallow. A typical description would be:
"Close your mouth, push your tongue to the roof, bite down, and swallow."
Direct physical manipulation in the form of jaw closure, digital pressure on
the base of the tongue to prevent tongue thrust, stroking of the laryngeal
area, lateral rocking of the larynx, application of digital pressure to the
sternal notch, and icing in an upward direction on the laryngeal area are
effective methods of stimulating a swallow. If patients begin the swallow but
do not complete it, it is frequently effective to either talk them through the
action, or to place an empty spoon back into their mouth, depress the tongue
and draw the spoon out, stimulating mouth closure around the spoon, and
thus start the swallow pattern again. The same can be done if feeding with a
syringe.

If patients have difficulty opening their mouths on command or in
response to food, do not force their chins open as this will cause increased
resistance. Instead, place your forefinger on the lower lip and pull down
gently. Another method is to tap the front teeth gently with a spoon. Many of
the patients who experience a pseudo-bulbar type of problem demonstrate
difficulty initiating and following through with the swallow. It is frequently
effective to go through the movements yourself as the patient does, instead of
describing what you want the patient to do. Words can frequently get in the
way. When patients are neurologically impaired and have significant com-

munication problems, visual cues throughout the swallowing process can be very helpful. One rule of thumb is to always try to simplify what you are doing with the patient, whether it is on a verbal or visual level or if you are physically manipulating the structures.

If patients are having difficulty swallowing liquids, begin with thick liquids; have them take a small sip, hold it in their mouths until they are "ready" to swallow, flex their heads forward, and swallow. This allows for better coordination of muscle movement and is frequently all the patient needs to take liquids efficiently. Sometimes, a routine of cough–swallow–cough–swallow or asking the patient to hold onto the swallow until the very end is helpful. Both of these techniques increase muscle contraction in the pharynx and at the level of the vocal folds. Helping the patient to visualize the swallow process may also be beneficial.

It is important that the patient's mouth be checked for any residual food before terminating therapy. Patients should remain in an upright position for 30 to 60 minutes after eating to reduce the chance that residual food stored in the pharynx or piriform sinuses can enter the trachea. A patient who experiences reflux due to an esophageal problem should remain in a sitting position for 60 minutes after eating.

Documentation of the amount and type of food swallowed is crucial in the management program. Caloric intake must also be recorded. This means you need to know exactly how much food or liquid you are giving a patient. Also important is to indicate the presence or absence of aspiration and then to measure the amount of food aspirated. The latter information is obtained when the patient is suctioned immediately following a feeding session. This kind of precision will allow for accurate assessment of progress.

In the initial stages of the treatment program the nurse may need to be present to suction the patient if there is any danger of aspiration. After each training session the nurse may be asked to assess the presence or absence of aspiration and to see that the patient remains upright for 30 to 60 minutes after eating. The amount of the next tube feeding needs to be adjusted according to the amount of oral intake.

When appropriate, the nurse carries out the training program at all meals and during administration of medication. The nurse and speech-language pathologist work closely in accomplishing this. The nurse also assists in training the family to take over feeding procedures, if necessary.

CONCLUSION

The complexity of the swallowing process and the type of intervention that is available reinforces the need for the dysphagic problem to be approached by a team of health professionals who can utilize their expertise in a coordinated manner. Programs such as these are highly successful in re-establishing an adequate swallow for oral intake—an essential function for the patient's physical and emotional well being.

Nurses play an integral role in the team effort to retrain the swallow in the brain-injured patient. Beginning with their initiation of the patient's referral to the dysphagia team, they maintain consistent involvement throughout the evaluation and treatment process, providing important information, medical supervision and expertise, and assistance in the direct training of the patient.

NOTES

[1]Evaluation forms can be obtained from the author.

[2]The term apraxia refers to difficulty initiating and completing a motor act on a voluntary level. The problem does not have to do with muscle weakness or spasticity but rather with the area of the brain that controls motor patterns.

ACKNOWLEDGMENT

This author gratefully acknowledges the assistance of Jeanine Pilario Brown, BS, RN, PHN, Director, Home Health Agency, Kaiser-Permanente Medical Center, San Rafael, CA, who acted as consultant in preparation of this chapter.

REFERENCES

Aliza, B.E. Dysphagia. Oral presentation at the Bay Area Group for Adult Communication Disorders, Kentfield, CA, March 15, 1979.

Aliza, B.E. Dysphagia in the neurologically impaired adult: Evaluation and therapy. Short course presented at the 28th Annual California Speech-Language-Hearing Association Conference, Los Angeles, March 28–30, 1980.

Brunner, L.S., & Suddarth, D.S. *The Lippincott manual of nursing practice* (2nd ed.). Philadelphia: J.B. Lippincott, 1978.

Buckley, J.E., Addicks, C.L., & Maniglia, J.E. Feeding patients with dysphagia. *Nursing Forum*, 1976, *25* (1), 69–85.

Burke Rehabilitation Hospital. *Treatment of dysphagia: A team approach.* Inservice training program presented at White Plains, N.Y. February 8, 1978.

Darley, F.L., Aronson, A.E., & Brown, J.R. *Motor speech disorders.* Philadelphia: W.B. Saunders, 1975.

Dobie, R. A. Rehabilitation of swallowing disorders. *American Family Physician*, 1978, *17* (5), 84–94.

Emerick, L.L., & Hatten, J.T. *Diagnosis and evaluation in speech pathology.* Englewood Cliffs, NJ: Prentice-Hall, 1974.

Fust, R.S. Dysphagia. In M. Skelly (Ed.), *Glossectomee speech rehabilitation.* Springfield, IL: Charles C. Thomas, 1973.

Gaffney, T.W., & Campbell, R.P. Feeding techniques for dysphagic patients. *American Journal of Nursing*, 1974, *74* (12), 2194–2195.

Gallender, D. *Eating handicaps: Illustrated techniques for feeding disorders.* Springfield IL: Charles C. Thomas, 1979.

Gray, H. *Anatomy of the body* (29th ed.). Edited by C.M. Goss. Philadelphia: Lea & Febiger, 1973.

Griffin, K.M. Swallowing training for dysphagic patients. *Archives of Physical Medicine and Rehabilitation*, 1974, *55*, 467–470.

Hargrove, R. Feeding the severely dysphagic patient. *Journal of Neurosurgical Nursing*, 1980, *12* (2), 102–107.

Hurwitz, A.L., Nelson, J.A., & Haddad, J.K. Oropharyngeal dysphagia. *Digestive Diseases*, 1975, *20* (4), 313–324.

Johnson, C.A., & Johnson, C.K. *Analysis of swallowing function in severe brain injury.* Paper presented at the Annual American Speech-Language-Hearing Association Conference, Houston, TX, 1976.

Langley, J., & Darvill, G. *Procedures for facilitating improvements in swallow, mastication, speech, and facial expression where these have been impaired by cerebral or peripheral nerve damage.* A manual prepared for undergraduates at the National Hospitals College of Speech Sciences. Hampstead, London: 1979.

Larsen, G.L. Conservative management for incomplete dysphagia paralytica. *Archives of Physical Medicine and Rehabilitation*, 1973, *54* (4), 180–185.

Larsen, G.L. Rehabilitation for dysphagia paralytica. *Journal of Speech and Hearing Disorders*, 1972, *37*, 187–194.

Mysak, E.D. *Neuroevolutional approach to cerebral palsy and speech.* New York: Columbia University, Teachers College Press, 1973.

Robins, V. Adkins, H.V., Linquist, J., Lim, V.J., & Dail, C.W. Physical therapy techniques for bulbar poliomyelitis. *The Physical Therapy Review*, 1958, *38* (8), 523–535.

Roueche, J.R. *Dysphagia: An assessment and management program for the adult.* Minneapolis: Sister Kenny Institute, 1980.

Seaman, W.B. Pharyngeal and upper esophageal dysphagia. *Journal of the American Medical Association*, 1976, *235* (24), 2643–2646.

St. Jude's Hospital and Rehabilitation Center. *Protocol for swallowing evaluation and treatment.* Presented at California Association of Rehabilitation Facilities Conference at San Francisco, March 23, 1981.

Winstein, C. Analysis and management of swallowing dysfunction. In *Rehabilitation of the head injured adult.* Downey, CA: Rancho Los Amigos Hospital, Professional Staff Association, 1980.

Zemlin, W.R. *Speech and hearing sciences: Anatomy and physiology.* Englewood Cliffs, NJ: Prentice-Hall, 1968.

8

Selecting and Implementing Augmentative Communication Methods for Adults

Donald L. Mast

INTRODUCTION

The necessity for the value of nurse-patient communication is well documented (Ashworth, 1978; LeRoux, 1977; Marsh, 1979; McGuire, 1979; McIntosh, 1979), however, certain disorders create barriers to effective verbal communication. This chapter deals with the problems of individuals for whom speech is not currently a functional means of meeting their communication needs. This includes both the temporarily and permanently nonoral adult and partially oral person who may or may not require augmentative communication systems.

A supplementary communication system may be necessary for individuals having the following disabilities: cerebral palsy (congenital); cardiovascular accident (aphasia), head trauma (acquired); amyotrophic lateral sclerosis and multiple sclerosis (progressive); certain postoperative conditions, and Guillain-Barré syndrome (temporary) (Vanderheiden, 1980). Additionally, treatment of deaf patients may require an interpreter in hospitals at no charge to the patient (Section 504 of the Rehabilitation Act of 1973).

The goal of habilitation or rehabilitation teams is to develop effective communication systems for nonspeaking persons (Vanderheiden, 1980) with maximal learning of or return of communication (DiSimoni, 1981). The intention throughout the chapter is to discuss nonoral communication in a manner applicable to adults and useful to the nurse in any setting. Augmentative refers to any device utilized to supplement communication.

COMMUNICATION SYSTEMS

DiSimoni (1981) suggests that alternate communication systems may be separated into the following categories: (1) communication boards, (2) mechanical communication devices, (3) nonspeech symbolic systems, (4) fingerspelling, (5) pantomime and gesture, (6) sign language, (7) intersystemic reorganization, and (8) biofeedback. Pantomime, intersystemic reorganization, and biofeedback will be omitted due to overlap and inapplicability to this discussion.

It is important to remember that nonoral communication is limited only by one's imagination (and sometimes budget!). Frequently, the simplest device or method can be effective. Subsequent to a review of the above named categories, special communication problems for the nurse will be discussed with suggested solutions and resources.

Communication Boards

Communication boards take a variety of shapes, sizes, forms, and content; however, they are typically easy and inexpensive to construct and can be tailored to the individual's needs and abilities. To illustrate, one need only survey the speech-language therapy unit in local hospitals to discover many have communication boards, binders, or alphabet boards prepared for use by patients. The commonality of message units needed by patients makes this feasible; however, in all nonoral communication systems one must be prepared to individualize the content.

The nonoral individual's skills, abilities, and needs, determined via a thorough assessment, will dictate how to prepare the best communication board. The *format* may range from notebook binders and ring binders of various sizes; message units mounted on lap boards (numerous styles are available), cardboard, or tag board; messages on 3 x 5 cards categorized and placed in a file box; messages placed on an easel near the patient; messages on a piece of cloth that can be folded and stored until required; or messages on plastic aprons for the ambulatory individual. The format of a communication board, simple or complex, will be dependent upon factors such as motor control, manual dexterity, visual abilities, mode of mobility, method of message indication, type and number of messages, and the amount of time this method of communication will be necessary.

An example of a format that is practical and inexpensive, yet an effective communication device that is easily constructed employs milk bottle caps mounted on velcro bracelets. These are primarily useful for the individual with limited motor abilities and capable of only a binary (e.g., yes/no) response. The caps can be placed on wrists, fingers, toes, or any body parts that are capable of gross, differentiating movements. "Yes/no," a happy/sad face, or some other appropriate set of messages are placed in the center of the bottle cap, with a gross movement of that body part sufficient to signal a response.

The *message units* on the communication board may be letters, numbers, words, phrases, pictures, nonspeech symbols, objects, photographs, or any other graphic depictions representing a message. If the individual has the skills necessary to construct sentences, the words should be organized in some systematic manner. Davis (1973) describes an adaptation for the non-oral individual of the Fitzgerald Key, designed for teaching language to the deaf. In this system, language is divided into the following categories and message units are placed and or organized according to these categories: who, what, where, and when words, and verbs. If the patient's language skills warrant, articles, conjunctions, prepositions, adverbs, and adjectives may be added. This system allows the contextual clues to supply the missing elements.

The Clarke School for the Deaf Language Curriculum Series (1972) provides a discussion and example of the Fitzgerald Key. (Clarke School for the Deaf, Northampton, MA.)

Communication boards are portable, allow the individual easy access to a means of communication, and are inexpensive. Limitations revolve around the fact that the audience must be present to receive a message and the style of a message unit may limit conversation to those who can read (word messages) or spell (alphabet board).

In developing the communication board, one should begin with a number of message units the patient can assimilate and gradually add messages. Ongoing monitoring with the necessary adjustments is vital. Changes in the board should reflect progression or regression in language development and or motor development, the change in communication needs (McDonald, 1975), or particular preferences expressed by the patient, family, or those with whom he or she continually communicates. It may be necessary to develop separate boards for different environments due to the variation in communicative requirements. For example, communications with a spouse, a nurse, a physical therapist, or friends would vary in terminology and content.

Regardless of the format, it is advisable to cover boards with clear contact paper or plexiglass, or to insert pages into plastic holders. This will protect the material from spills, drooling, and general wear and tear.

Individualization of communication boards is governed by certain basic elements, but can be an expanding process to maximize the individual's potential. Initially, one must consider the physical capabilities of the individual. If there appears to be limited range of motion, it would be advisable to evaluate the individual's ability to point to enhance the placement of messages. This can be accomplished by using a magic marker or crayon (or for individuals possessing only gross grasping ability, a crayon made by melting crayolas in muffin tins). In evaluating position, place the patient in his or her communication posture and place butcher paper on the area anticipated to be occupied by the communication board. The patient then marks on the paper, reaching limits both left and right, away from and close to the body. The message units can then be placed within these boundaries.

During the interview, the informant may provide information which will allow you to further personalize the communication board. Other individualizing factors include favorite phases the person may have previously utilized (e.g., "All right!," "Awesome!"); the opportunity to express frustration and anger (e.g., "Darn it!," or "Geez!"); names of family, friends, and pets; and adjustments in board content at the appropriate times of year to accommodate holidays and birthdays, seasons of the year, and events such as the baseball season.

Oakander (1980) provides a resource for implementation of language boards.

Mechanical Communication Devices

The sophistication of communication aids varies greatly, therefore, aid selection should be tailored to the individual's skills, abilities, and needs. The devices discussed here will demonstrate aids both commercially available and some that can be easily constructed.

The *clock face communicator* has some variations, although the basic form is a clock hand driven by an electric motor with the message units placed at intervals around the outside of the face (Luster & Vanderheiden, 1974). By activating the interface, the clock hand scans the available messages, with the individual stopping the hand when the desired message is reached. Messages are most useful when flexible; thus, using magnets or placing messages on hooks allows for easy adjustments. Suggestions for constructing such a device include use of a barbecue rotisserie motor or clock motor with the second hand utilized as the pointer. These motors may be mounted on an appropriately strong material to serve as the clock face on which the messages will be mounted.

The *communication roll* (Brieditis, 1974) is a cylinder within a cylinder with message units placed on the inner cylinder. A small window in the outer cylinder allows viewing of the message, with the inner cylinder turned by manipulating an attached wheel by hand, foot, or other means.

The *Etran Eye Signaling System* (Eichler & Neale, 1974) consists of a piece of plexiglass standing upright between the sender and receiver. An aperture at its center allows the individuals sending and receiving messages to view one another. Letters are placed at eight distinct areas on the glass, with the sender directing his or her eyes to one of the areas and the receiver speaking the selected letter. If correct, the receiver writes the letter on the message paper and returns the gaze to the sender for the next letter. This system can also employ a grid system of message units, with the sender's selections corresponding to the row and column of the message.

The *HandiVoice*, distributed by Phonic Ear, Inc., [1] utilizes speech to assist the nonoral individual in communicating. The individual touches the display board at the appropriate point to select words, phrases, speech sounds, and prefixes/suffixes. The words are produced aloud and combined into sentences by the device. Two models are available to accommodate varying physical and intellectual abilities with memory capabilities in both.

The *Canon Communicator*, distributed by Telesensory Systems, Inc., [2] is a portable communication aid utilizing a keyboard with a strip printer display. Entries include the alphabet, numbers, and a variety of punctuation marks.

The *Zygo Model 100 Communication System*[3] utilizes 100 light emitting diodes in a 10-by-10 matrix. Messages are placed on transparencies, and the Zygo has the ability to recall any 16 items in the order entered.

Although this is not an exhaustive list of mechanical communication devices, it does provide examples of the three modes of output (visual, printed, and speech) and the three approaches to message selection (scanning, encoding, and direct selection) previously discussed.

For a more complete resource, see the annotated bibliography of communication aids (Luster & Vanderheiden, 1974), or the photographs and discussion provided by Jones (1981).

Fingerspelling/Sign Language

Fingerspelling is a system of communication utilized primarily by the deaf and hard-of-hearing to supplement sign language. Each letter of the alphabet has a corresponding hand configuration (Watson, 1972). Because of the tedious and time-consuming nature of spelling every word of a communication, it is seldom used as a sole means of communication. Additionally, the movements for fingerspelling require a certain level of fine motor control, thus limiting the population for whom it is useful. It is imperative that the audience know fingerspelling so messages can be understood.

There are numerous recognized sign language systems, among which are Seeing Essential English (SEE₁); Signing Exact English (SEE₂); Amerind; Paget-Gorman Sign System (PGSS); and American Sign Language (ASL or Ameslan). SEE₁ and SEE₂ utilize a syntax that parallels spoken and written English (Mayberry, 1976). Ameslan is telegraphic in its messages, omitting articles and lacking differentiation between he, she, it, and pronouns in nominative and accusative cases. Some ASL signs do not have spoken English counterparts and vice versa. Amerind is a gestural code based on the "hand talk" of the American Indians. Researchers (Skelly, Sehinsky, Smith, & Rust, 1974) report a high rate of understanding even by untrained receivers. PGSS is a signing system which mirrors spoken English, including every part of speech, prefixes, and suffixes.

As with any nonoral communication system, selection of a signing (manual communication) system will depend on the situation, need, and the particular patient (DiSimoni, 1981). Selection of a manual communication system will also be influenced by the style of preference for a given geographical location. As with fingerspelling, however, the patient's manual dexterity/fine motor control and the receptive signing skill or willingness of those in the individual's environment to learn a sign system will be necessary considerations.

Gestures

From one society and culture to another there exist gestures that carry common meaning. An experience that most of us have had is to require assistance of someone who speaks a different language. We immediately resort to gestures to aid in communicating. This serves to illustrate that almost without exception we each possess a moderate *gestural vocabulary*. Since the guidelines consist of making gestures as concrete and universal as possible, the remainder is up to the individuals communicating.

It is helpful if everyone attempting to communicate with the individual uses the same gestures. A sample list of gestures suitable for adults to supplement a communication system is included in Table 8-1.

TABLE 8-1

Gestures to supplement verbal and nonverbal communication

NOTE: Many of the concepts presented may have to be taught. Gestures should be as concrete and universal as possible. Whenever possible, have the individual determine or assist in determining the gesture for a concept. Add or delete gestures as needed.

up	point up, look up
down	point down, look down
in	fingertips enter "O" formed by other hand
out	opposite of in
on	palm of one hand is placed *on* other hand or some item
over	hand arches *over* other arm
under	hand slides *under* other arm
sick:	
stomachache	palm of hand on stomach
headache	palm of hand on forehead
hot	hand wipes brow or fans face
cold	arm(s) wrap around body as if trying to keep warm
come here	beckon with index finger or whole hand
go away	palm out, pushing away
I'm hungry	palm of hand circles against stomach
I'm thirsty	pretend to drink from a glass
sleepy	lay head on hand(s) forming a pillow
What?	palms up, shrug
Where?	shake index finger from side to side
When?	take index finger in a circle, tracing a clock in the air
we	alternately point to another individual and then self
you, your	point to other individual
me, my, I, mine	point to self
tall, big	hand measures *tall*
short, little	hand measures *short* or thumb and index finger approximate *short*
yes	head gesture
no	head gesture
listen	cup hand to ear
look	index finger moves from eye to pointing at object to be looked at

TABLE 8-1 (continued)

more .... whole hand beckons as in *come here*, but
                        many times
quiet .... index finger to lips, i.e., *sh*
today, now .... point emphatically straight down
tomorrow, later .... index finger arches forward
yesterday, earlier .... thumb or index finger motions behind self

COMMUNICATION SYSTEMS: OVERVIEW

Prior to discussing the various methods of nonoral communication, some components common to numerous systems will be reviewed. These components will then be utilized when discussing the systems.

Interfaces

The *interface* is that portion of a system with which a person interacts to make the device work (Coleman, Cook, & Meyers, 1980); in essence it is the control. Coleman et al. (1980) use examples of the keyboard on an electric typewriter and the light switch's relationship to a light as excellent illustrations of interfaces in our daily lives. A key element in assessing the nonoral client is to determine a behavior the client can voluntarily, reliably, and consistently control. Given today's technology, any reliable, consistent response can be utilized to operate a communication device.

Some interfaces utilize common movements and incorporate simple strategies, while others harness movements that surprise the novice. One common used control is called the *joy stick*, which resembles a gear shift in a sports car, and is frequently seen as the control on electric wheelchairs. The joy stick may be operated conventionally with the hand, or via head control with the assistance of a cup-like receptical which houses the chin. A pointer or wand can be attached to a helmet or head harness (*head pointer*) or mounted in a bite plate (*mouth stick*), thus head control is utilized. Variations of levers (*rock lever*), paddles (*paddle switch*), and buttons are employed for the patient to depress. *Mercury switches*, activated by tipping or tilting, can be positioned on any appropriate portion of the body. *Pneumatic switches* are operated by very small pressure changes and can be activated by sipping or puffing.

Other switches that rely on the aforementioned technology include: *touch switches*, activated by touching a prescribed sensor area with any skin surface; *moisture sensitive switches*, activated by contact with the tongue; *proximity switches*, activated by bringing a certain body part within a certain range of the switch; *optical switches*, utilizing a beam of light attached to some part of the body, which is used to operate photosensitive switches on a panel; *sonic switches*, activated by a predetermined sound; and *bioelectric switches*, utilizing the application of electrodes to the skin near a controllable muscle group. A thorough review of these and other interfaces is included in Vanderheiden and Grilley (1975).

These examples serve to emphasize the importance of the evaluation activities. It is essential to determine the method of control to maximize the individual's language skills and abilities, rather than underestimate the patient's abilities. A communication device needs to take advantage of optimum communicative potential.

Evaluation may reveal the need to modify certain features of a communication system. One area to consider is the patient's reaction time in utilizing a control switch and his or her ability to cease the movement once the desired message has been achieved. Some devices are manufactured with selectors to set the time allowed for a response. For example, the patient's depression of a switch causes a light to move across a matrix at a speed of 1 square per second until the desired message is achieved. If this is too rapid for the patient's reaction time, the selector can be reset so the light moves at a rate of 1 square every 10 seconds (or some desired delay).

Assistive devices are also available to facilitate communication efforts. An individual may possess the necessary range of motion and accuracy to point as a means of selection, but require the assistance of a plastic splint with an extending appendage to hold in his or her clenched fist (Griffin & Gerber, 1980).

Approaches to Message Selection

Regardless of the employment of interface, there are three primary approaches to selecting a message. These approaches are scanning, encoding, and direct selection, or some combination of the three (Vanderheiden, 1980). In *scanning*, the communication device or the individual with whom one is communicating points to the message items until the nonoral person indicates the correct item has been reached. A simple example is *yes/no* questioning until the correct question is posed. *Encoding* utilizes two or more code elements which specify the message element. An example of this method would have messages in a grid format with the columns and rows designated by numbers. The nonoral individual selects the two numbers corresponding with the desired message. In *direct selection*, the individual points directly to the desired message. A common example would be a language board with pictures depicting messages to which the nonoral person points.

Message Units

Message units for communication boards and mechanical communication devices can consist of letters, numbers, words, phrases, pictures, nonspeech symbols, objects, photographs, or any other graphic depiction representing a message. Three symbol systems will be elaborated on here: Bliss Symbols, Rhebus, and Non-speech Language Initiation Program (Non-SLIP).

The Bliss Symbol System, developed by Charles Bliss (1965), consists of an alphabet of 100 basic symbols, 30 currently recognized worldwide (e.g., punctuation, Arabic numerals, mathematical signs). Two or more symbols are combined to form new concepts. Bliss Symbols are pictorial (e.g., ↑ for tree), ideographic (e.g., ♡ to represent the abstract concept of a feeling), or arbitrary (e.g., from a recognized symbol as — for a part of). Each symbol may signify a number of related meanings (e.g., ⌂ may be interpreted as *house* or *building*, depending on the context in which it occurs. Bliss Symbols and information on this nonspeech symbol system may be obtained from: Blissymbolics Center, Loma Linda University, Loma Linda, CA 92354.

Rhebus symbols, initially developed to assist in teaching reading, are pictures representing words. Subsequently, a Rhebus system has been developed for use as a communication system (Kiernan, 1980).

Non-SLIP, developed by Joseph Carrier and Timothy Peak (1974), utilizes nonspeech symbols formed by plastic chips. Each chip is unique in shape and color, with the program being designed for individuals for whom oral language training has failed. The primary emphasis is to reduce the complexity of language training by developing a visual array of nonspeech symbols (Carrier, 1974).

Selection of the style of message unit to be utilized should be tailored to the needs, skills, and abilities of the nonoral person. Input from the nonoral individual regarding his or her preferences is important.

Output

Communication aids provide three modes of output: visual, printed, and speech. *Visual* output is illustrated by a communication board which the receiver must observe to obtain the message. *Printed* output can be either hard or soft copy. Hard copy relates to communicators that provide a printed record of the communication, e.g., strip printer/ticker tape. Soft copy refers to an alpha-numeric keyboard which produces message units on a light-emitting diode display (DiSimoni, 1981). *Speech* output refers to devices utilizing tape recorded messages or synthetic speech output.

Bigge and O'Donnell (1976) specify the advantages of the various output systems. Visual output is effective in a person-to-person communication.

Printed output allows for storing and sending of information for later use. Speech output allows for interchange with others and gives the nonoral individual a psychological boost. Montgomery (1980) cites further advantages of visual output, including high visibility, flexibility of displays, and editing capabilities. Additional values of printed output systems are permanency, ability to include punctuation, allowance for long-distance correspondence, and the fact that they are designed around commonly recognized symbol systems (Montgomery, 1980).

Selection of message units and a mode of output for a patient must consider numerous variables, most notably the ability to read, the ability to process information, and skill in implementing a sequence of directions. Typically, the adult's skill levels in these areas would be well-known; thus, assessment can focus on detection of any deficiencies resulting from disease, surgery, or other trauma.

THE IMPORTANCE OF THE NURSE

The importance of the nurse with the non- or limited-oral patient centers on the continual patient contact. The practical nature of the nurse-patient intercourse, the opportunity to observe and glean information regarding the patient's communication needs and abilities, and the opportunity to provide information to family, doctors, speech-language pathologists, and other professionals regarding potential modifications in the mode or system of communication place the nurse in a position to assist in maximizing the patient's communication abilities. Areas in which the nurse's involvement and input are valuable are:

(a) *Initially*—Assisting the speech-language pathologist with identification through differential diagnosis and observation and or referral to the speech-language pathologist.

(b) *In the home*—Providing assistance/support to spouses and other members of the family; monitoring quantity/quality of communication; suggesting modifications to facilitate improved communication.

(c) *In the hospital*—Assisting with assessment, communication "practice," and suggesting modifications in mode and or system of communication; referring; providing input on communication needs (including message units).

(d) *Before and after surgery*—Referring post-surgical patients whose previously identified communication system/mode is no longer appropriate or may need modification(s). Preoperative training and orientation with potential nonoral communication methods are essential.

(e) *Health team*—Providing input regarding health status and prognosis of the nonoral individual.

(f) *For referral*—Evaluating communication skills for adequacy and effectiveness.

(g) *Rehabilitation process*—Encouraging the patient to utilize communication skills maximally; monitoring; providing feedback regarding the patient's changing skills (physical, oral) evidenced in the patient and further communication needs (message units).

REACTIONS AND RESISTANCE TO NONORAL COMMUNICATION

Self-concepts of the patient and reactions of the family and others to the non- or limited-oral individual or augmentative communication systems vary; however, common problems can be anticipated. The person's mental capacity is sometimes questioned (Creech, 1981; Viggiano, 1981). There are expectations that time, medical care, and love will resolve the problems and the patient's status will return to normal. Other priorities such as orthopedic problems may preempt the expenditure of time, money, and effort on communication issues. An environment that does not require the individual to assume a communicative role creates dependence and reduces the need to develop or utilize the patient's own communication skills. The family or others can react with pity for the person and his or her plight. The nonoral individual and those interacting with the patient typically feel frustrated at the time, effort, and difficulty required during communication situations normally taken for granted. The family's anger for reasons already stated or expressed by searching questions (e.g., "Why did this happen to me?") may dampen the enthusiasm for communication. A general attitude of defensiveness prevails for the nonoral person's situation. An attempt may be made by family and friends to deal with the communication problem without professional speech help due to a lack of credibility for that professional, the inaccessibility of a qualified professional, or lack of funds for such service. This may lead to more frustration and resistance due to the unsatisfactory progress in communication.

In dealing with resistive factors, it is important for the team members planning nonoral communication to assure resistive individuals that nonoral, alternate, or augmentative communication systems are not and should not always be considered a last resort or a sign of failure, i.e., a negative prognosis for speech (McDonald & Schultz, 1973). In fact, with a nonoral communication system, an individual is usually less tense, and therefore able to vocalize more easily (McDonald & Schultz, 1973).

Vanderheiden (1980) notes that many persons have reservations regarding the use of nonspeech techniques unless traditional techniques have failed. He states that such reservations are unfounded and can result in delayed communication development or delay the development of intelligible speech.

The nurse should be aware of these potential misconceptions and concerns and be prepared to contend with them. This can be accomplished by providing support to the patient and his or her family, directing them to such resources as literature and other professionals, and taking the time to listen to concerns.

Shane (1981) provides answers to questions typically posed regarding augmentative communication systems.

NEEDS OF THE NONORAL POPULATION

The non- or limited-oral individual needs an effective (Vanderheiden, 1980) and immediate (DiSimoni, 1981) means of communication. From a practical viewpoint, one's desires and needs must be expressed. These include biological needs, daily communicative give-and-take, social needs, and the opportunity to maintain dignity, if only through the ability to communicate.

Losses or deficits of the person who does not have the ability to communicate by conventional means include:

(a) The loss of ability to initiate and determine the direction of conversations (McDonald & Schultz, 1973). This leads to a dependence on others for communicative necessities and puts the individual at the "communicative mercy" of others.

(b) Reduced language development and organization of vocabulary, syntactic and morphologic rules, and concepts (DiSimoni, 1981; Vanderheiden, 1980; Harris-Vanderheiden and Vanderheiden, 1977).

(c) Reduced development of skills in organizing ideas and thinking (McDonald & Schultz, 1973).

(d) Reduced development of social (Vanderheiden, 1980), emotional, and intellectual/academic skills (Griffin & Gerber, 1980; McDonald & Schultz, 1973; Vanderheiden, 1980).

(e) Frustration and anger due to continual misinterpretations and oversimplifications of needs and underestimations of intellect and personality.

These losses can be minimized and the person's needs met through an effective communication system. The presence or absence of these and other communicative symptoms noted by nurses, speech-language pathologists, and other team members may be clarified or substantiated by the team during the evaluation.

EVALUATION CONSIDERATIONS

Major Goals of Assessment

The major goals in assessing the nonoral client are to determine current levels of development and to match the communication needs and situational constraints of a speech and language prosthesis to these levels (Coleman et al., 1980; DiSimoni, 1981).

Appropriate Communication System Selection

The election of an appropriate communication aid or the decision to delay or reject (Shane & Bashir, 1980) an augmentative communication system relies on a thorough evaluation, preferably by a multidisciplinary team. The composition of this team may vary depending on the work setting, the age and client type, and the professionals available.

Coleman et al., (1980) cite the cooperative efforts of biomedical engineers, psychologists, and speech-language pathologists as productive in The Assistive Device Center at California State University, Sacramento. More commonly in settings where the intent is not to develop new communication aids, but to select an aid currently available, a team may consist of medical personnel (nurse/doctor), speech-language pathologist, physical therapist/occupational therapist, teacher, and parent or spouse.

The Nurse's Role in Team Evaluation

The nurse's responsibilities on the assessment team will vary with the team composition. The nurse will be able to provide input on the individual's health status in relation to the overall program of rehabilitation. The nurse may make the initial referral to the team for consideration of a nonoral evaluation and make home visits or conduct interviews to gather additional data. Also, because of the continuous nature of their contact with the patient, nurses in the hospital can monitor and report changes in physical and mental status, the varying affects medication may be having on the individual, and the effectiveness of communication. When difficulties arise, the nurse can be a vital link in the team's problem solving system.

Because of the nurse's knowledge of the patient, he or she can provide recommendations regarding modifications in the interface, message units, or output system of the communication process, suggest intervention regarding the individual's attitude toward nonoral communication, or call on the appropriate professional to resolve a particular problem. The nurse may also advise other staff members on the patient's communication needs and methods. This will facilitate continuity of communication for the nonoral patient. The nurse can serve as the team member who interfaces with all other disciplines.

Common Components of Assessment

Common elements are evident in determining an individual's current levels of performance and communication needs with the intent of selecting an augmentative communication system. The person's physical status, including motor abilities, sensory factors, and mode of mobility greatly influence the mode of operation, selection of an interface, and the physical attributes of the device. An estimate of the patient's cognitive abilities will directly relate to numerous factors regarding complexity of operation, symbol system, and language level. Communication skills and needs have an obvious relationship to the decisions made in device selection.

An underlying consideration in evaluation of the nonoral individual is that assessment tools have not yet been normed on this population. Assessment results,then, must be weighed with this in mind. When evaluation results present a questionable picture, professionals working with nonoral persons typically give the individual the benefit of the doubt. It is better to err in this direction than underestimate the patient's potential.

Additionally, the environment into which a sometimes expensive, delicate device is to be taken, must be evaluated. Consider the home setting, the communication that occurs in this environment, and the involvement and cooperation espoused by the family. Has equipment previously been provided this individual? How well has it been maintained? This may assist in appraising the readiness of those in the home environment for accepting responsibilty for care and use of a nonoral communication device. A list of factors regarding evaluation of the home environment is included in Table 8–2.

TABLE 8–2
HOME VISIT
Related factors concerning nonoral communication

HOME SETTING

Type of dwelling: apartment; single-family house; other _____

Family group consists of _____

Frequent house guests   Yes   No   Frequency of visitors _____

Adaptations previously made in the home environment _____

_____

Adaptive equipment (present or past) _____

Condition _____ How long have they had it? _____

Source from which it was borrowed _____

House size—could individual signal need to communicate from room to

room?   Yes   No   Method of signing _____

What appliances does the individual operate independently, e.g., TV, radio,

phone? _____

Is the individual mobile at home?   Yes   No   Type of mobility (include

whether typically on the floor or in wheelchair) _____

Percentage of time for each _____

COMMUNICATION

Who communicates with the individual at home? _____

TABLE 8–2 (continued)

Amount of time spent communicating daily _____

Method of communication _____

Effectiveness _____

Is frustration evident regarding communication? Yes No   If so, for

whom _____ Comment on the reverse side

what elements of communication create most frustration, e.g., amount,

method, limitations. Need for additional communication at home — a

little; moderate amount; great deal. How much does the patient get out

(besides school) where communication would be used? _____

INVOLVEMENT/COOPERATION

How involved is the spouse/family likely to be? _____

What can be expected to be carried out at home? _____

Recent Research

Various authors and researchers have proposed strategies for evaluating the nonoral individual. Vanderheiden (1980) has developed a "Parallel Profile" approach to evaluation and communication system recommendation. The profile consists of two columns, one containing the user (patient) evaluation components and the other an aid evaluation profile. The user evaluation and the parallel aid evaluation components are shown below:

User Evaluation

Physical
Cognitive
Communication and control
  needs/constraints

Aid Evaluation

Physical and operational
Cognitive/comunication aspects
Communication and control
  capabilities

Assessment of the subcomponents of the user (patient) evaluation categories provides information regarding the individual's needs, capabilities, and limitations. When applied to the aid (device) capabilities, a profile of the appropriate communications/control system capabilities is obtained.

Coleman et al. (1980) gather information via interviews and assessments. Interviews are conducted regarding functional skills (medical history and sensory and motor abilities), communication skills (receptive and expressive language), and device utilization (where and how the aid is to be used, amount of time to be used, packaging, arrangement, portability, and type of copy). A task analysis follows, which provides information concerning the necessary behaviors the individual must perform and the communication tasks the device is to facilitate. Assessments are then conducted to determine current levels of physical and language performance.

Shane and Bashir (1980) utilize a decision matrix consisting of 10 factors; cognition, oral reflex, language, motor-speech, speech intelligibility, emotional, chronological age, response to previous therapy, ability to imitate, and environmental factors. Analysis of each factor utilizes a branching index to yield a decision to elect, delay, or reject implementation of an augmentative communication system.

In noting that an effective communication system includes specific and clearly understood interactions, Griffin and Gerber (1980) concur with Harris-Vanderheiden and Vanderheiden (1977) when they state that these interactions develop from an accurate assessment of cognitive skill levels, receptive language, expressive language, speaker-listener interaction (pragmatics), and an analysis of immediate and long-range needs. The authors above also consider motivation to communicate, prognosis for effective oral communication, physical and social environments, primary audience, visual and auditory abilities, and method of mobility as important factors to evaluate.

In response to the increasing complex decisions required to pair a nonoral communication system to the skills and needs of an individual, Beukelman and Yorkston (1980) rely on a two-phase assessment, combining a capability-need evaluation and a performance evaluation. The initial portion of the assessment involves motor, intellectual, visual-perceptual and linguistic capabilities, and communication needs. The latter phase consists of assessing the nonvocal communicator's use of a particular system in a variety of communication environments.

In summary, it is important to regard assessment as ongoing (Harris-Vanderheiden & Vanderheiden, 1977), as typically, cognitive, language, and physical abilities and skills will change over time, as will the person's communication needs. Thus, a communication system must be dynamic (Harris-Vanderheiden & Vanderheiden, 1977; McDonald, 1975) and keep pace with the nonoral individual's development. Similarly, when a progressive disease causes deterioration in a patient's cognitive, language, and or physical status, the communication system must be appropriately modified. Nurses' daily activities place them in a prime position to monitor change in the physical and mental status of an individual, to evaluate the effectiveness of communication provided by a nonoral device, and to recommend modifications to enhance communication.

SPECIAL COMMUNICATION PROBLEMS FOR THE NURSE

Some individuals suddenly find themselves without the ability to communicate due to a medical problem. Special communication problems will be discussed, with resources for additional information and possible solutions the nurse may implement.

Stroke Patients

The individual who has suffered a cerebral vascular accident can present many and varied speech and language problems. The nonoral systems previously discussed may be appropriate for this individual. Ford (1978) provides a brief, but useful, list of nursing guidelines for working with aphasic patients.

DiSimoni (1981) demonstrates the utilization of Bliss symbols with the aphasic patient.

Intubated Patients

Individuals who require lifesaving devices such as endotracheal or tracheostomy tubes experience an inability to communicate vocally, which frequently creates feelings of isolation and fear (Lawless, 1975). Because this situation is usually temporary, time-consuming communication aid development or large expenditures are not necessary. Simple use of pad and pen, Magic-Slate, gestures, visual aids, a flip-chart booklet, language cards, artificial larynx (Walker, 1979; Lawless, 1975), or a vocabulary/alphabet board (Blomefield, 1978) would be effective. Helping the patient understand the treatment provided, implications of that treatment, and keeping lines of communication open will help reduce his or her anxieties and fears.

See Presley (1980) for an excellent example of how a tracheo-
tomized patient utilizes gestures, pantomiming, and signaling
systems.

Intensive Care Unit (ICU)

Patients in ICU frequently understand the necessity for certain health care
procedures but are not able to comprehend the physical limitations imposed
by them. These patients may not understand the medical terminology and
jargon utilized by the team members. Nonoral persons have the same basic
physical needs of verbal patients in ICU. Nonoral patients need to be able to
express their physical needs, such as "pain" or "suction me" (Lawless, 1975).
It is important that one of the techniques discussed in this section or in the
section on communication systems be employed to reduce frustration and
fear when the nonoral patient is in ICU.

Ashworth (1978) discusses "communication in the intensive care
unit."

Disease and Accidents

Head trauma, and at times disease (e.g., Guillain-Barré, amyotrophic
lateral sclerosis), will not only reduce or eliminate patients' communication
abilities, but may leave them almost completely immobile. A nurse may have
to be imaginative and go beyond "one eye blink for 'yes' and two blinks for
'no'" to develop a system to meet these patients' capabilities. See Chapter 6
for further discussion of head trauma.

Schreiber (1979) gives an interesting account of a nursing staff's
ingenuity in solving a patient's communication problem.

Limited/Non-English-Speaking (LES/NES)

The non-English-speaking patient may have capabilities in his or her
native language; however, in an English-speaking environment this patient

may manifest certain symptoms of the nonoral individual. Although obvious and real, the LES/NES individual's problems are not considered a communication disorder as defined in this book. In emergency situations, however, nonoral communication methods will be required.

Depending on the circumstances, the person may respond to: (1) gestures, (2) bilingual communication boards (with the English counterpart for the nurses's benefit), or (3) an interpreter on staff. A list of available individuals who may provide assistance is essential.

Perron (1976) provides guidelines for nurses' communication with non-English-speaking and deaf patients.

Deaf and Hard-of Hearing

Section 504 of the Rehabilitation Act of 1973 requires hospitals to provide at no cost to the patient, interpreter services to deaf patients. Navarro and LaCourt (1980) feel a staff should be able to gain information by having the patient write, by asking him or her to "show me," or the staff should learn a few useful signs. Additionally, these authors provide some guidelines for communication with the deaf and hard-of-hearing, some emergency signs, and the fingerspelling alphabet. Curry (1980) discusses methods of communicating with this population. Sabatino (1976) provides a lengthy list of suggestions for deaf patient care while Jensen (1976), Mulrooney (1976), and Wolf (1977) provide numerous suggestions for using interpreters, background on the emotional status of the deaf patient, and information concerning some of the particular needs of this population. For a thorough discussion of deafness, see Chapter 4.

The Registry of Interpreters for the Deaf, P.O. Box 1139, Washington,DC 20013, local public schools, college, university, or club for deaf individuals have names of qualified interpreters.

Laryngectomy

Many of the methods discussed in this chapter may be of assistance to the laryngectomee. Various alaryngeal procedures, taught by a speech-language pathologist, are provided in Chapter 2.

RECOMMENDATIONS FOR THE NURSE

Nurses, in complementing the work of speech-language pathologists, need certain information to make themselves more effective as members of the rehabilitation team.

Nurses should:

1. Be aware of the referral source(s) and the referral process. The nurse may have the earliest and most convenient opportunity to informally assess the individual's communication skills, and initiate a referral through the appropriate channels.

2. Develop a basic knowledge of the elements and concerns regarding assessment of the nonoral individual given above. Realize the role and responsibilities the nurse has as a member of the multidisciplinary team in the work setting.

3. Keep abreast of developments in nonvocal communication systems and their components, including interfaces, approaches to message selection, message units, output modes, and some of the various types of communication systems.

4. Become aware of various community resources that might assist in developing and constructing communication aids, including the Pioneers of America (retired telephone workers), high school and college vocational classes, senior citizens' groups, and local handimen. (Contact the local telephone company or consult a resource guide of community organization for existence and location of groups.)

5. Become familiar with funding sources, for example, Medicare, Regional Centers, Department of Vocational Rehabilitation, and philanthropic organizations, e.g., Elks, Lions, Kiwanis.

6. Encourage your professional library to subscribe to *Communication Outlook*, a practical publication on nonoral communication systems selection, implementation, and development (Artificial Language Laboratory, Computer Science Department, Michigan State University, East Lansing, MI 48824).

7. Be aware of local resources and facilities dealing with assessment and dispensing of nonoral communication systems. Local resources may include public school speech-language pathologists, speech-language pathologists in private practice, speech-language pathologists working in hospital clinics, and communicative disorders departments at colleges and universities. Appendix 8–1 lists facilities that deal with nonoral communication devices and systems.

CASE STUDY AND RATIONALE FOR
SELECTION AND IMPLEMENTATION
OF NONORAL COMMUNICATION DEVICES

Note: The following case study is an actual case; however, the identifying data have been changed to protect the identity of the individual.

Case: E.K., a middle-aged man with amyotrophic lateral sclerosis, a degenerative neurological disease, was referred from a college clinic. Upon initial contact speech was still relatively intelligible, but the expectation was a relatively rapid loss of functional speech. Confined to a wheelchair, and dependent on others for mobility, E.K. delighted in conversing with friends, his wife, and sons. Motor abilities were still relatively good, including arm movement, manual dexterity, upper torso, and head control.

Even when speech was still a useful means of communication, a sentence construction board was developed with E.K.'s help. The board was made on tag board, covered with clear contact paper, mounted on a light wooden frame, and placed on E.K.'s lap board. Instruction in the communication board's use began immediately, even though it would be some time before it was required.

Gradually E.K. began to tire towards the end of the day, so the board was used. He would point to the message units (words, some phrases) and the receiver would say the words, frequently anticipating the conclusion of the sentence to save E.K. time and energy. Letters were also present, so words not on the board could be constructed. After some time speech was no longer intelligible, and the motor abilities of his arms began to decrease. Communication became laborious, tiring, and frustrating. At that point an alphabet board was constructed with the letters forming a slight arc from left to right. E.K. was fitted with a head pointer and with good head control could rapidly spell out messages.

At the same time a concern came from his wife that their evening conversations took forever to get through with very little content. To alleviate this problem, another head pointer was procured and tailored to utilize with an electric typewriter. Now, while his wife was at work, E.K. could type paragraphs of "conversation" or type letters to family members. Evening conversations then utilized the paragraphs as focal points to facilitate communication.

As left to right head movement decreased, the 26 letters of the alphabet were divided into two rows of 13 letters forming a chevron. Subsequently, E.K. could no longer sit upright in his wheelchair and was confined to bed. E.K. resorted to eye blinks to respond "yes" or "no" to questions while the next alternative in providing a means of communication was considered. A board on the ceiling above E.K.'s bed was to be developed, with a light source replacing the head pointer. However, prior to this modification, E.K. died.

Two important lessons were learned in this case. Nonoral communication systems are dynamic, ever-changing. Team members must be alert to changes in physical and communication skills and needs. Secondly, E.K.'s family made a critical point: They were thankful for his ability to live his last months with dignity and purpose through the ability to continue effective communication.

Reactions From Consumers and Professionals

The feelings of two consumers who have benefitted from nonoral communication devices were recently published in a journal of the American Speech-Language-Hearing Association (Creech, 1981; Viggiano, 1981). Creech (1981) sees speech as the most important sense, with a detrimental effect on one's psychological and sociological development noted when verbal interaction is absent or limited. Creech (1981) suggests that people talk to and not about, the nonoral person. As long as the general public is uncomfortable with the nonoral population, the consumers feel they will continue to be ignored socially, and misconceptions about physical limitations will abound. Creech (1981) also states that effective communication is the only means to create the understanding which will erase these misconceptions and prejudices.

The American Speech-Language-Hearing Association has recently drafted a position statement on appropriate intervention for nonspeaking persons and points to the responsibility of speech-language pathologists to educate coworkers in this area of communication augmentation (Ad Hoc Committee on Communication Processes and Nonspeaking Persons, 1981).

The intent of this chapter is to provide nurses with a knowledge base that will enhance the treatment provided the nonspeaking person. Because of the rapid advances in the development of augmentative communication techniques, there is no nonspeaking person too handicapped to benefit from some type of augmentative communication system (Ad Hoc Committee on Communication Processes and Nonspeaking Persons, 1981).

NOTES

[1]HC Electronics, Inc., 250 Camino Alto, Mill Valley, CA 94941

[2]3408 Hillview Ave., P.O. Box 10099, Palo Alto, CA 94304

[3]Zygo Industries, P.O. Box 1008, Portland, OR 97207

ACKNOWLEDGMENT

This author gratefully acknowledges the assistance of Sarah Greene, BA, RN, Staff Nurse, Emergency Department, Merced Community Medical Center, and Instructor of Nursing, Merced College, Merced, CA, who acted as consultant in preparation of this chapter.

REFERENCES

Ad Hoc Committee on Communication Processes and Nonspeaking Persons. Position statement on nonspeech communication. *Asha*, 1981, *23*, 577–581.

Ashworth, P. Communication in the intensive ward. *Nursing Mirror,* February 1978, pp. 34–36.

Beukelman, D.R., & Yorkston, K.M. Nonvocal communication: Performance evaluation. *Archives of Physical Medicine Rehabilitation*, 1980, *61*, 272–275.

Bigge, J.L., & O'Donnell, P.A. *Teaching individuals with physical and multiple disabilities.* Columbus, OH: Charles E. Merrill, 1976.

Bliss, D.K. *Semantography—blissymbolics.* Sydney, Australia: Semantography Publications, 1965.

Blomefield, J. A vocabulary board for communicating with patients. *Respiratory Care*, 1978, *23*, 290–291.

Brieditis, K. Communication roll. In M. Luster & G. Vanderheiden, *Annotated bibliography of communication aids.* Madison, WI: Cerebral Palsy Communication Group, 1974.

Carrier, J. Non-speech noun usage training with severely and profoundly retarded children. *Journal of Speech and Hearing Disorders*, 1974, *17*, 510–517.

Carrier, J., & Peak, T. *Non-speech language initiation program.* Lawrence, KS: H&H Enterprises, 1974.

Coleman, C., Cook, A., & Meyers, L. Assessing non-oral clients for assistive communication devices. *Journal of Speech and Hearing Disorders*, 1980, *45*, 515–526.

Creech, R. Attitude as a misfortune, *Asha*, 1981, *23*, 550–551.

Curry, J. The hearing impaired patient: Stranger in a strange land. *ETHICON*, 1980, pp. 18–20.

Davis, A. Linguistics and language therapy: The sentence construction board. *Journal of Speech and Hearing Disorders*, 1973, *38*, 205–214.

DiSimoni, F.G. Therapies which utilize alternative or augmentative communication systems. In R. Chapey (Ed.), *Language intervention strategies in adult aphasia.* Baltimore: Williams & Wilkins, 1981.

Eichler, J.H., & Neale, H.C. *Etran eye signaling system.* In M. Luster & G. Vanderheiden, *Annotated bibliography of communication aids.* Madison, WI: Cerebral Palsy Communication Group, 1974.

Ford, M. Communicating with the aphasic patient. *The Journal of Practical Nursing,* 1978, *28,* 20–21.

Griffin, H., & Gerber, P. Non-verbal communication alternatives for handicapped individuals. *Journal of Rehabilitation,* 1980, *46,* 36–39.

Harris-Vanderheiden, D., & Vanderheiden, G. Basic considerations in the development of communicative and interactive skills for non-vocal handicapped children. In E. Sontag (Ed.), *Educational programming for the severely and profoundly handicapped.* Reston, VA: Council for Exceptional Children, 1977.

Jensen, D. The silent minority. *Nursing,* October 1976, p. 15.

Jones, D. Computers revolutionize aids for nonspeakers, *Asha,* 1981, *23,* 555–557.

Kiernan, C. The hands say it. *Nursing Mirror,* September 1980, pp. 16–20.

Lawless, C. Helping patients with endotracheal and tracheostomy tubes communicate. *American Journal of Nursing,* 1975, *12,* 2151–2153.

LeRoux, R. Communicating with the dying person. *Nursing Forum,* 1977, *16,* 145–155.

Luster, M., & Vanderheiden, G. *Annotated bibliography of communication aids.* Madison, WI: Cerebral palsy Communication Group, 1974.

Marsh, N. The patient needs to talk. *Nursing Mirror,* 1979, pp. 16–18.

Mayberry, R. If a chimp can learn sign language, surely my non-verbal client can too. *Asha,* 1976, *18,* 223–228.

McDonald, E. Design and application of communication boards. In G. Vanderheiden & K. Grilley (Eds.), *Non-vocal communication techniques and aids for the severely physically handicapped.* Baltimore, MD: University Park Press, 1975.

McDonald, E., & Shultz, A. Communication boards for cerebral palsied children. *Journal of Speech and Hearing Disorders,* 1973, *38,* 73–88.

McIntosh, J. The nurse-patient relationship: Communication with patients. *Nursing Mirror*(Suppl.), January, 1979, pp. 148:i-ii+.

McGuire, M. Storm signals. *Nursing,* 1979, *9,* 136.

Montgomery, J. *Non oral communication: A training guide for the child without speech.* Non Oral Communication Project, Exemplary/Incentive Dissemination Project, Title IV-C, ESEA, 9675 Warner Ave., Fountain Valley, CA 92708, 1980.

Mulrooney, J. Deaf-patient care: A special concern to me. *RN,* June 1976, pp. 69–70.

Navarro, M., & LaCourt, G. Helpful hints for use with deaf patients. *Journal of Emergency Nursing*, November/December 1980, pp. 26–28.

Oakander, S. *Language board instruction kit*. Non Oral Communication Project, Exemplary/Incentive Dissemination Project, Title IV-C, ESEA, 9675 Warner Ave., Fountain Valley, CA 92708, 1980.

Perron, D. Nursing implications. *Nursing Digest*, Summer 1976, p. 42.

Presley, S. When it comes to communicating without words...Cyrus was an expert. *Nursing*, October 1980, pp. 82–85.

Sabatino, L. Do's and don'ts of deaf-patient care. *RN*, June 1976, pp. 64–68.

Schreiber, C. To communicate with Mrs. Savage, we put bells on her toes. *Nursing*, March 1979, pp. 47–49.

Shane, H. Working with the nonspeaking person: An interview with Howard Shane. *Asha*, 1981, *23*, 561–564.

Shane, H., & Bashir, A. Election criteria for the adoption of an augmentative communication system: Preliminary considerations. *Journal of Speech and Hearing Disorders*, 1980, *43*, 408–414.

Skelly, M., Sehinsky, L., Smith, R., & Rust, R. American Indian Sign (Amerind) as a facilitator of verbalization for the oral-verbal apractic. *Journal of Speech and Hearing Disorders*, 1974, *39*, 445–456.

Vanderheiden, G. Augmentative modes of communication for the severely speech- and motor-impaired. *Clinical Orthopedics and Related Research*, May 1980, pp. 70–86.

Vanderheiden, G., & Grilley, K. *Non-vocal communication techniques and aids for the severely physically handicapped*. Baltimore, MD: University Park Press, 1975.

Viggiano, J. Ignorance and handicap. *Asha*, 1981, *8*, 551–552.

Walker, C. Ultimate frustration: The intubated patient. *RN*, September 1979, pp. 118b+.

Watson, D. *Talk with your hands*. Winneconne, WI: 1972.

Wolf, E. Communicating with deaf surgical patients. *AORN Journal*, 1977, *1*, 39–46.

APPENDIX 8-A

Some facilities that conduct research, assess, and or develop nonoral communication devices

This partial list will serve as a resource for centers where one may receive services, or where one may be referred to consultants or agencies in a specific geographical location. A portion of this listing comes from a compilation by Judy Montgomery (1978), Non-Oral Communication Center, Fountain Valley, CA. Information regarding locations of and services provided by facilities can also be obtained from the Artificial Language Laboratory in Michigan.

ALABAMA

Program: Regional Blissymbolics Resource Center

Contact Person: Pam Elder

Address: DESEMO Project
P.O. Box 313
University Station
Birmingham, AL 35294

CALIFORNIA

Program: Rehabilitation Engineering Center

Contact Person: Margaret Barker

Address: Children's Hospital at Stanford
520 Willow Road
Palo Alto, CA 94304

Program: Non-Oral Communication Center

Contact Person: Judy Montgomery

Address: 9675 Warner Avenue
Fountain Valley, CA 92708

Program: Assistive Devices Center

Contact Person: Collette Coleman

Address: California State University, Sacramento
6000 J Street
Sacramento, CA 95819

Program: Blissymbolics Center

Contact Person: Mel Cohen

Address: Loma Linda University
Loma Linda, CA 92354

Program: Northridge Hospital Foundation

Contact Person: Pam Schiffmacker

Address: 18300 Roscoe Blvd
Northridge, CA 91324

Program: United Cerebral Palsy Center—San Diego

Contact Person: Nancy Oro

Address: 7947 Birmingham
San Diego, CA 92123

MARYLAND

Program: Rehabilitation Department

Contact Person: Barbara Sonies

Address: National Institutes of Health
Bethesda, MD 20014

MASSACHUSETTS

Program: Biomedical Engineering Center

Contact Person: Rick Foulds

Address: Tufts New England Medical Center
Rehabilitation Institute
171 Harrison Avenue
P.O. Box 1014
Boston, MA 02111

MICHIGAN

Program: Artificial Language Laboratory

Contact Person: John Eulenberg

Address: Computer Science Department
Michigan State University
East Lansing, MI 48824

NEBRASKA

Program: Meyer Children's Rehabilitation Center

Contact Center: Faith Carlson

Address: University of Nebraska Medical Center
444 South 44th Street
Omaha, NB 68131

NEW JERSEY

Program: Cerebral Palsy Association of Middlesex County

Contact Person: Travis Tallman

Address: Roosevelt Park
Edison, NJ 08817

TENNESSEE

Program: Rehabilitation Engineering Center

Contact Person: Elaine Trefler/ Doug Hobson

Address: University of Tennessee
1248 La Paloma Street
Memphis, TN 38114

WASHINGTON

Program: Department of Rehabilitation Medicine

Contact Person: David Beukelman

Address: University Hospital
BB919 RJ-30
Seattle, WA 98195

WISCONSIN

Program: Trace Center

Contact Person: Gregg Vanderheiden

Address: 1500 Johnson Drive
University of Wisconsin—Madison
Madison, WI 53706

APPENDIX
Library Resources

Vicky Christianson

A supplemental list of research tools that may be found in most libraries is given below. Another excellent method of searching the literature is MED-LINE (MEDical Literature Analysis and Retrieval System on-LINE) developed by the National Library of Medicine. An article by Barbara J. Reiner and Christy L. Ludlow entitled "Using MEDLINE for literature retrieval in the communicative disorders" (*Asha*, 1981, *23*, 655–662) will explain how to use that source.

RESOURCES

Bibliography of developmental medicine, and child neurology; books and articles received. London: Spastics International Medical Publications in association with William Heinemann Medical Books, 1958 —

Child development abstracts and bibliography. Washington, D.C.: National research council, etc., 1927 —

Cumulated Index Medicus. Chicago: American Medical Association, National Library of Medicine, 1960 —

Cumulative Index to Nursing and Allied Health Literature. Glendale, CA: Glendale Adventist Medical Center, 1956 —

Current index to journals in education. New York: CCM Information Sciences, 1969 —

DSH abstracts. Danville, IL: Deafness Speech and Hearing Publications, American Speech and Hearing Association, 1960 —

Developmental disabilities abstracts. Washington, D.C.: Developmental Disabilities Office, 1964–1978.

The Education Index. New York: The H.W. Wilson Company, 1930 —

Educational Resources Information Center. Catalog of selected documents on the disadvantaged. Washington: U.S. Government Printing Office, 1966.

Exceptional child education resources. Reston, VA: Council for Exceptional Children, 1969 —

LLBA: Language and language behavior abstracts. Ann Arbor: Sociological Abstracts, Inc., 1967 —

Language—teaching and linguistics: abstracts. London: Cambridge University Press, 1963 —

Psychological Abstracts. Lancaster, PA: American Psychological Association, 1927 —

ACKNOWLEDGMENT

   This contributor would like to gratefully acknowledge the assistance of Mr. Bill Heinlen, Head, Reference Department, California State University, Fresno, Henry Madden Library, who acted as a consultant in the preparation of this appendix.

Author Index

Subject Index